This book belongs to:

_____

Presented by:

_____

Date:

_____

THE WARRIOR

There was a time when all was well
It all seems easier, looking back,
But hardships only time would tell,
Were readied for attack.

It's never easy to find out
What's going on inside,
It's never easy to learn about
How we'll face the raging tide.

Perhaps you felt nothing wrong,
Perhaps you suffered every day,
And you felt scared all along,
The diagnosis was on its way.

All of a sudden, the clock counts down,
Decisions coming hard and fast,
And you are looking all around,
Hoping it will make sense at last.

We all must take a different path,
We're all facing our own beast,
For each a different aftermath,
We have each other, at least.

We cannot give in, or stand alone,
Even though hope might fade.
With every ounce of blood and bone,
Must fight even when we're afraid.

Perhaps the light at the end shines bright,
Perhaps we've done all we can do,
And yet with all our summoned might
We shall be carried through.

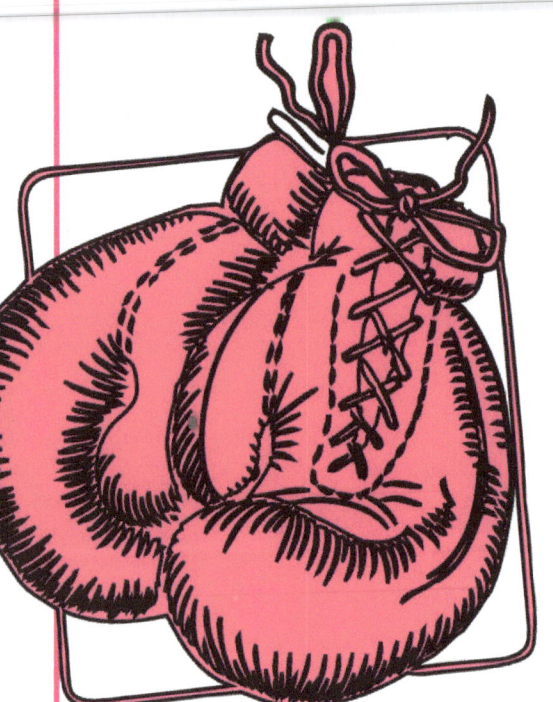

I, _____ **am a Warrior!** *The Fight is Real* **& I am more than a conqueror!**

B.O.P CANCER
The Fight is Real

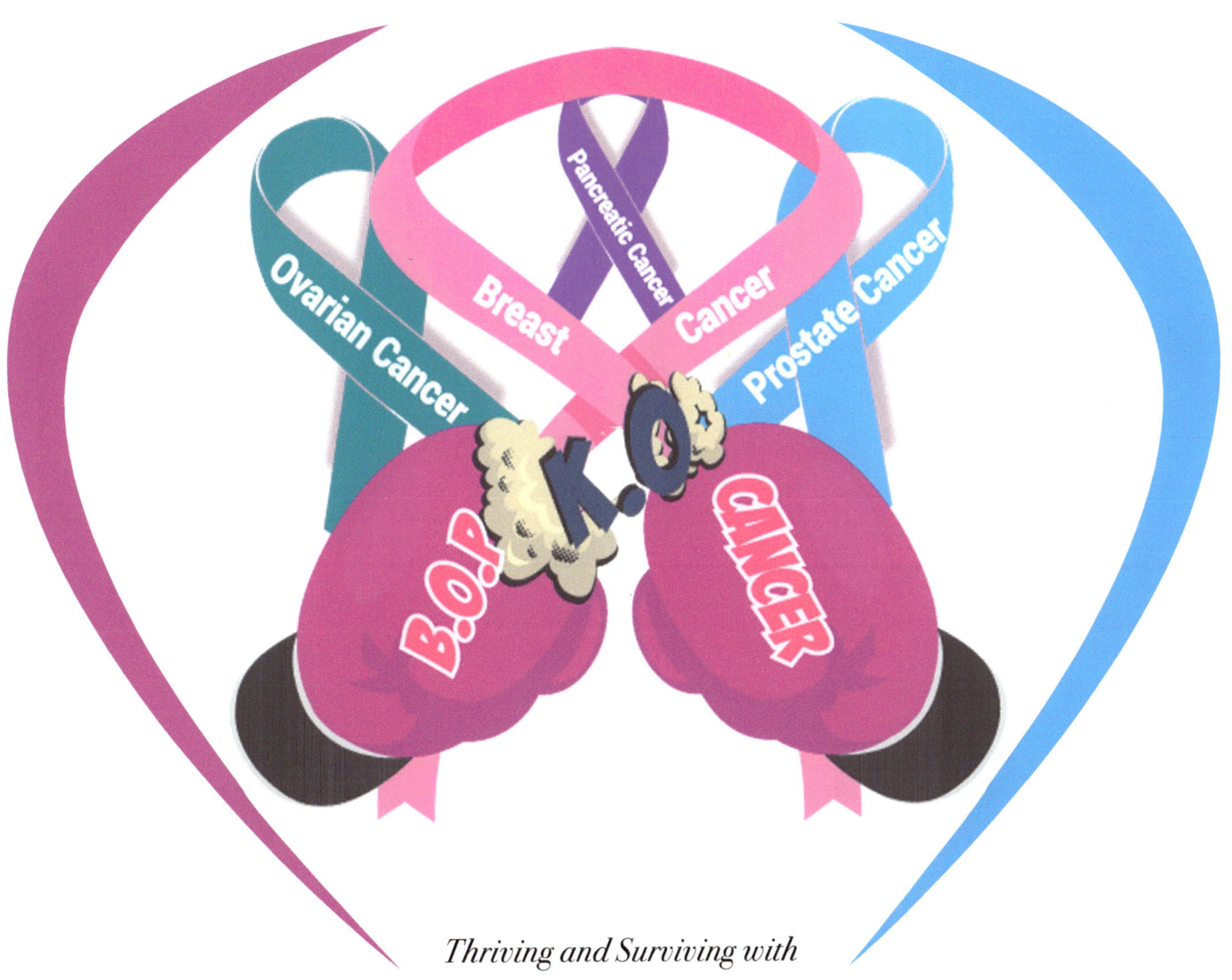

*Thriving and Surviving with
mental awareness and inspirational activities*

Breast Cancer- Series I

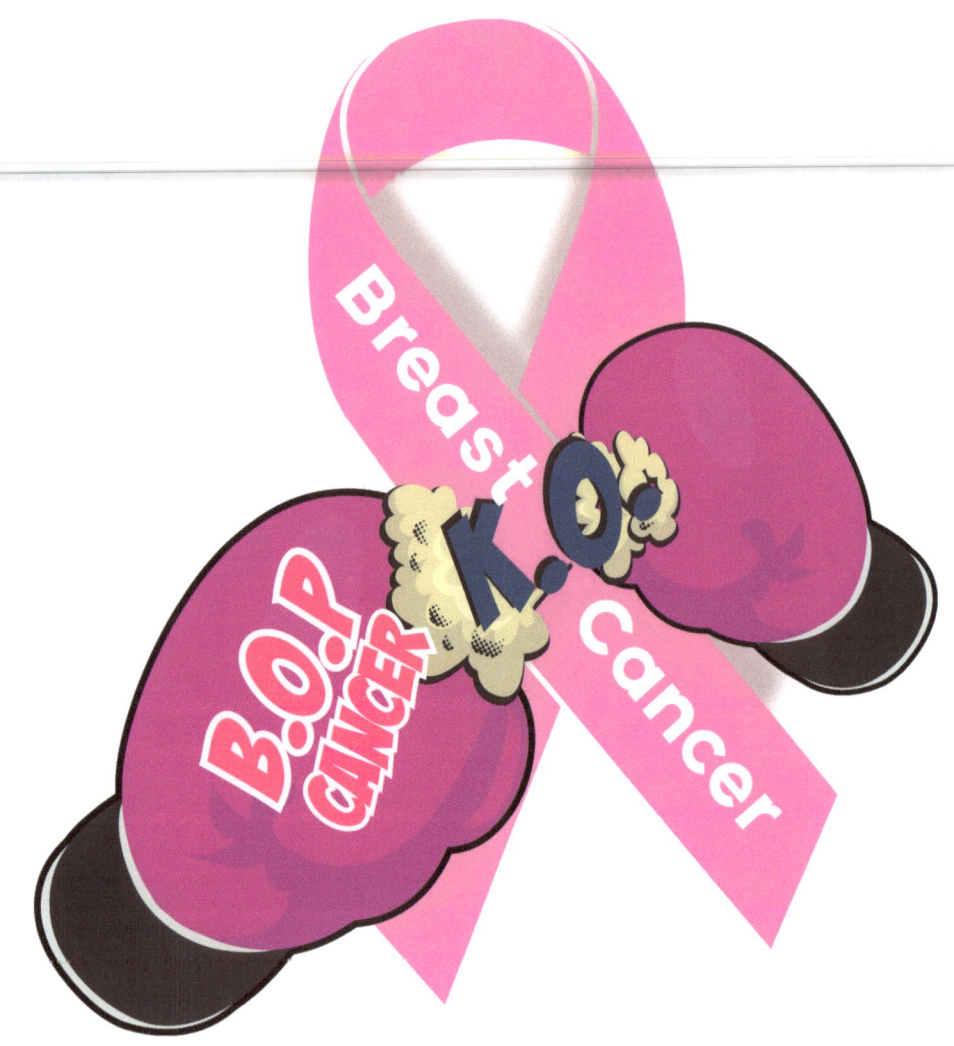

April L. Jones, PhD

April Jones, PhD

B.O.P. Cancer- The Fight is Real:
Thriving and Surviving through Mental Awareness and Inspirational Activities.
Copyright ©2018 by Dr. April L. Jones.
All Rights Reserved.
No part of this publication may be reproduced in any form whatsoever, by photography or photocopied or any other means, stored in a retrieval system, by broadcast or transmission, by translation into other languages, nor by recording electronically or otherwise, without prior written permission from the author except by a reviewer, who may quote brief passages in critical reviews or articles; or authorization through payment of the appropriate fees to the
Copyright Clearance Center, Inc., 222 Rosewood Drive, Danvers, MA 01923, 978-750-8600,
Info@copyright.com or on the web at www.copyright.com

Published by Visionary Consulting Services, LLC
www.vcsllc.co
Cover/Design: Kreashuns Graphics Group
ISBN-13: 978-1986062138

ISBN-10: 1986062139
BISAC: Medical/Mental Health/Cancer
Library of Congress Control Number:2019905593
CreateSpace Independent Publishing Platform
North Charleston, SC
Printed in the United States of America.

Disclaimer:

The information provided in this book is designed to provide helpful information on the subjects discussed. This book is designed to provide information and motivation to our readers. It is sold with the understanding that the publisher and author is not engaged to render any type of psychological, legal, or any other kind of professional advice. This book is not meant to be used, nor should it be used, to diagnose or treat any medical condition. For diagnosis or treatment of any medical problem, consult your own physician. The publisher and author are not responsible for any specific health needs that may require medical supervision and are not liable for any damages or negative consequences from any treatment, action, application or preparation, to any person reading or following the information in this book.

No warranties or guarantees are expressed or implied by the publisher's choice to include any of the content in this series. Neither the publisher nor the individual author shall be liable for any physical, psychological, emotional, financial, or commercial damages, including, but not limited to, special, incidental, consequential or other damages. Our views and rights are the same: You are responsible for your own choices, actions, and results.

References are provided for informational purposes only and do not constitute endorsement of any websites or other sources. Readers should be aware that the websites listed in this book may change.

DEDICATION

This book is dedicated in loving memory of my cousin, Whitney Charday Jones, who passed away from triple negative breast cancer. Also, in memory of Major T. Danielle Russell, who too passed away from triple negative breast cancer. Your love and cheer is missed, but your fight is to be replicated by all who face cancer.

"Those who leave us leave their legacy, it is a mantle we must carry forward." - Dr. Jones

The 413 Foundation was set up by Dr. Albert E. Russell to honor his late wife, Dr. Tomeka D. Russell. The name is derived from the date of her passing, April 13th and also from Danielle's favorite scripture, Philippians 4:13 "I can do all things through Christ who strengthens me." The Dr. Tomeka D. Russell Scholarship Fund provides financial assistance to female, African-American students from the states of Alabama, Florida or Georgia who plan to attend medical school. Students must be enrolled in a university and may be Freshmen-Senior classification. For more information visit https://www.tdrlegacy.com/about/

HONOREES

This book honors those who have BOP breast cancer and giving back by sharing their stories. Women and Men of true strength who have painted the picture of hope to a fighter of breast cancer.

In honor of:
Mrs. Cynthia Holt, 3 time survivor of 17 years
Mrs. Aloys Ingram, 1 time survivor of 19 years
Ms. Lawanna Barron, 1 time survivor of 7 years
Mr. Leafus Taylor, 1 time survivor of 6 years

"The brave act of survival, day by day, sparks endless hope in others." - Dr. Jones

BOOK REVIEW

In order to understand the basic premise of *B.O.P. Cancer: The Fight is Real*, a different approach to cancer management, it is first necessary to receive the definition of 'B.O.P' which Dr. Jones provides in the opening introduction of her book: *"B.O.P Cancer is the slang expression for knocking out (K.O.) cancer."* Why 'B.O.P'? It also serves as an acronym from the four types of cancer addressed in the book series (Breast, Ovarian, Prostate, and Pancreatic cancers).

The focus is on mental awareness and care routines, with *B.O.P. Cancer* filling in many gaps in cancer literature by providing a self-help psychological inspection of approaches to cancer's mental and physical challenges and how to overcome them.

This strategy is, of necessity, multifaceted. After a brief introduction (which prior patients will already know, but those newly diagnosed might need) of cancer's types, diagnoses, stages, treatments and causes, Jones moves to the meat of her discussion: traversing stages of grief, employing mentally stimulating puzzles and exercises to distract and strengthen mental acuity, resilience, and positive thinking, and covering all aspects of psychological self-help.

The spiritual is not neglected during this process: readers receive sections about spirit animals, mantras, and other exercises and reflections which include plenty of fill-in invitations for self-help, as well as Biblical passages.

There is no singular approach or focus to this book, which calls upon all tools from traditional to new age to address the ravages of dealing with cancer.

It's this wider-ranging approach than most which gathers a plethora of resources under one cover, offering cancer patients and their caretakers a workbook that serves as a template for positive emotional and spiritual reinforcement.

It's a motivational guide that shares stories, compiles routines and approaches that work, and generally injects comfort and peace into a chaotic situation.

Cancer patients and their caregivers need to make this toolkit a part of their arsenal for positive paths away from negativity, overwhelm, and chaos.

-D. Donovan, Senior Reviewer
Midwest Book Review

TABLE OF CONTENTS

Dedication — 7

Honorees — 8

Book Review — 9

Introduction — 12

Breast Cancer Awareness — 15

Color Comfort — 22

Poetry — 46

Puzzles — 50

Affirmations, Intentions, Inspirational Quotes — 60

Humor — 67

Spirit Animals	71
Inspirational Scriptures	92
Mindful Mediations	96
Useful Websites	103
Appendix	104
(Puzzle Answers, Self Exam Chart, Signs of Cancer Chart)	
About the Author	114
Retail Store	115
B.O.P Series & Album	117

INTRODUCTION

What does B.O.P. Cancer Mean?

B.O.P Cancer is the slang expression for knocking out (K.O.) cancer. In this book reader's will find ways to bop cancer by learning about the type of cancer, causes, treatment, mental awareness, and enjoy some of the self-help activities that may reduce psychological stress of cancer fighters' and caregivers to a person living with cancer. The focus of the book is mental wellness through information and relaxing activities. B.O.P. Cancer is also unique in wording because it is an acyronym from the four types of cancer addressed in the book series, which are Breast, Ovarian, Prostate, and Pancreatic Cancers

Cancer Overview

The human body consists of billions of small cells that form different organs and tissues. Our blood cells, bone cells, skin cells, muscle cells, and all other organs are built up of these small cells. They have a range of functions - the blood transports oxygen and substance through our body, the skin protects our body, lungs allow oxygen to be taken into the body while enabling the body to get rid of carbon dioxide, and so on.

Throughout life, old cells die and get replaced with similar cells through cell division. Millions of cell divisions happen in the human body every hour and if any defective cells are formed, they get destroyed by our immune system.

Cancer is a consequence of a disturbance in the balance of normal cell division – when the cell division continues even after it should have stopped and grows into surrounding tissues. Eventually, the cancer cells form small lumps, tumors that grow and spread.

Today, there are more than 200 different types of cancer. According to National Cancer Institute, 39, 6% of people will get cancer in their lifetime. However, thanks to modern research, many people are cured.[1]

Cancer and Mental Awareness

A cancer diagnosis may have a weighty impact on person's mental health. If you are fighting cancer, it is not unusual to experience mental health distress. Whether you are coping with the cancer diagnosis, the challenges of treatment, or constant worry about a recurrence, emotions triggered by the cancer experience can be hard to handle.

Cancer may bring on a variety of emotions, including (but not limited to) disbelief and shock, fear, anxiety, sadness and grief, depression, anger, low self-esteem, and feelings of helplessness.

FIGURE 1- Stages of Emotions

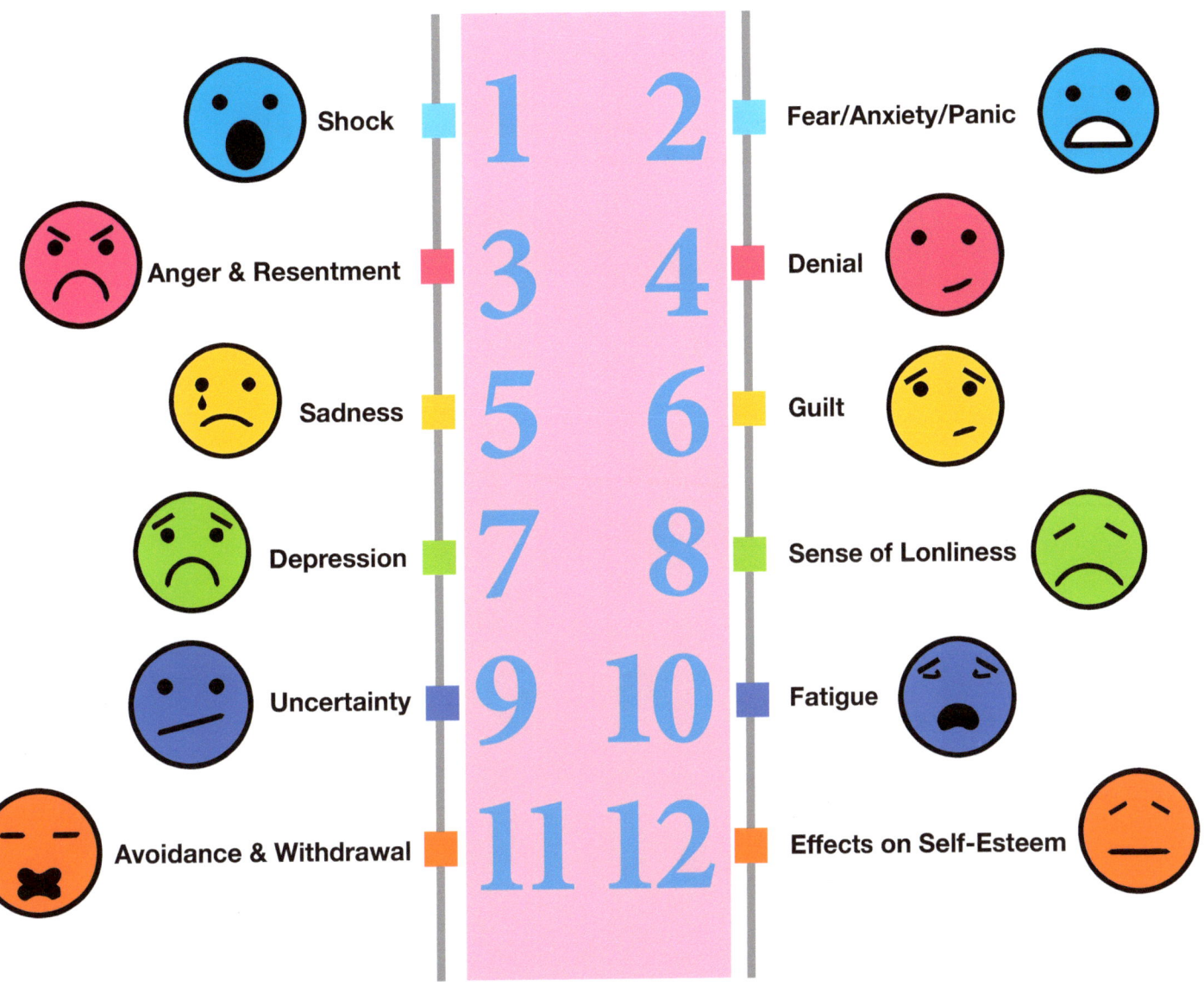

Thus mental wellness care is necessary and an integral part of cancer care. Addressing your psychological well-being can help you feel more relaxed and in control, cope better with the treatment, overcome anxiety and depression, and enjoy life.

In this book, you will find useful tips and information about mental wellness and self-help practices for people fighting B.O.P (breast, ovarian, prostate and pancreatic) cancer and their caregivers. The main aim of this book is to raise awareness about the importance of psychological well-being when fighting and/or caring for someone with B.O.P. cancer.

For further information, please visit
https://www.cancercenter.com/community/managing-side-effects/emotional-psychological/
https://www.mesotheliomagroup.com/our-mission/resources/mental-health/

---

[1] National Cancer Institute, "Cancer Statistics", Last updated March 22nd 2017, https://www.cancer.gov/about-cancer/understanding/statistics

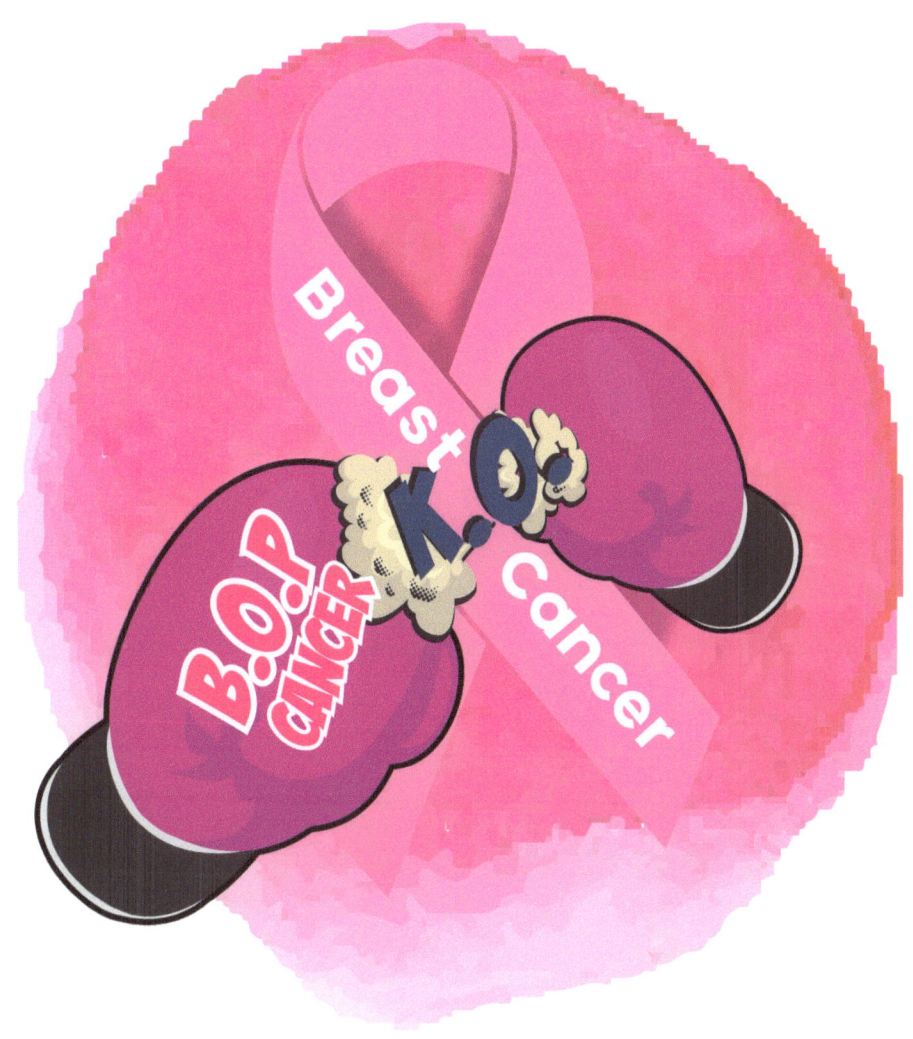

Breast Cancer Awareness

After non-melanoma skin cancer, breast cancer is the most frequent malignancy diagnosed in women worldwide. According to the U.S. National Cancer Institute, more than 230,000 women and 2,600 men in the United States get diagnosed with breast cancer each year.

Breast cancer can occur in both women and men. However, it is far more common in women.

Male breast cancer forms in the breast tissue of men. Although is most common in older men, it can occur at any age. Breast cancer is cancer that forms in the cells of the breasts. Nowadays, breast cancer survival rates have increased, mainly due to such factors such as a better understanding of the disease, early detection and a new personalized approach to treatment. [2]

Breast Cancer Types

- Inflammatory breast cancer
- Angiosarcoma
- Ductal carcinoma in situ (DCIS)
- Paget's disease of the breast
- Male breast cancer
- Recurrent breast cancer

Signs and symptoms

Make an appointment with your doctor for an evaluation if you notice any of the following, as it may be signs of breast cancer:

- A breast lump
- A thickening that feels different from the surrounding tissue
- Change in the appearance, size or shape of a breast
- An inverted nipple
- Dimpling or other changes to the skin over the breast
- A nipple discharge
- Redness or pitting of the skin over the breast
- Peeling, scaling, flaking or crusting of the pigmented area of skin surrounding the areola (nipple)

Causes

Breast cancer occurs when some breast cells begin to grow abnormally and divide more rapidly than healthy cells. They finally form a lump or a mass and can spread (metastasize) to other parts of the body.

Researchers have found that different genetic, hormonal, lifestyle and environmental factors and their interaction, may increase the risk of the breast cancer. It is estimated that about 5 to 10 percent of breast cancers are linked to gene mutations passed through generations of a family.

Breast Cancer Prevention

Integrating the following routines into a lifestyle may reduce the risk of breast cancer.

- ✓ Screenings
- ✓ Self-exams
- ✓ Regular exercise
- ✓ Maintaining a healthy weight
- ✓ Choose a healthy diet

BRCA Gene Test

Women who are likely to have an inherited mutation in either one of the two breast cancer susceptibility genes — BRCA1 and BRCA2 have an option of undergoing BRCA Gene Test. This test uses DNA analysis to identify harmful mutations in either of these two genes.

Women with inherited mutations in BRCA1 and BRCA2 genes are at an increased risk of developing breast cancer and ovarian cancer compared with the general population.

Treatment

The doctor determines the breast cancer treatment based on the type of the breast cancer, its size, stage, and grade, taking into consideration patient's own preferences and their overall health. The treatment may include surgery, radiation therapy, chemotherapy, hormone therapy, and supportive care.

Breast Cancer and Mental Health Issues

The link between breast cancer and psychological health is well documented. Mental disorders brought on by breast cancer affect the patient's normal functioning and are among the leading causes of disability worldwide.

The most common psychological outcomes in breast cancer patients and survivors are the following:

- Shock and disbelief
- Uncertainty and fear
- Sadness and grief
- Guilt
- Anxiety
- Depression
- Frustration and anger
- Feelings of isolation
- Low self-esteem and feelings of vulnerability

According to a study published online in August 2017, the prevalence of depression among women who had breast cancer ranged from 10 to 20 percent.

Breast cancer and its treatment can cause a range of feelings that are very hard to cope with. For example, after mastectomy, a great number of women experience feelings of damage, depreciation in the value of their body, hopelessness, and reduction in attractiveness. These feelings can further lead to different mental disorders.

According to one study, most of the women that underwent mastectomy struggled with a low body-esteem that affected their overall mental health. [3]

During breast cancer treatment many women find themselves overwhelmed with many different emotions such as fear, worry, uncertainty, sadness, and grief. It is important to know the stages of grief to recognize this emotion and the cycle of 5 stages of grief. The stages of grief are denial, anger, bargaining, depression, and acceptance.

5 STAGES OF GRIEF

DENIAL
The person refuses to accept the realty of the situation.
"This can't be happening to me."

ANGER
The person gets angry with themselves, or those around them.
"I've never smoked a cigarette in my life. How could this happen to me!"

BARGAINING
The person tries to strike a deal with God in attempt to reach compromise. "If my test comes out clear, I'll quit smoking for the rest of my life."

DEPRESSION
The person begins to accept the situation but this is accompanied by sadness. "I give up. Its not like I can do anything about it."

ACCEPTANCE
The person begins to accept the situation and recognize that the illness is going to impact their life. "Yes, this is happening to me."

FIGURE 2

These emotional issues may arise after treatment as well. In addition, women with breast cancer face other challenges, such as changed physical appearance after breast cancer surgery or sexuality after breast cancer.

Considering the significant role mental health factors play in patients' overall well-being, it is vital that a psychological support becomes an integrated part of comprehensive cancer care.

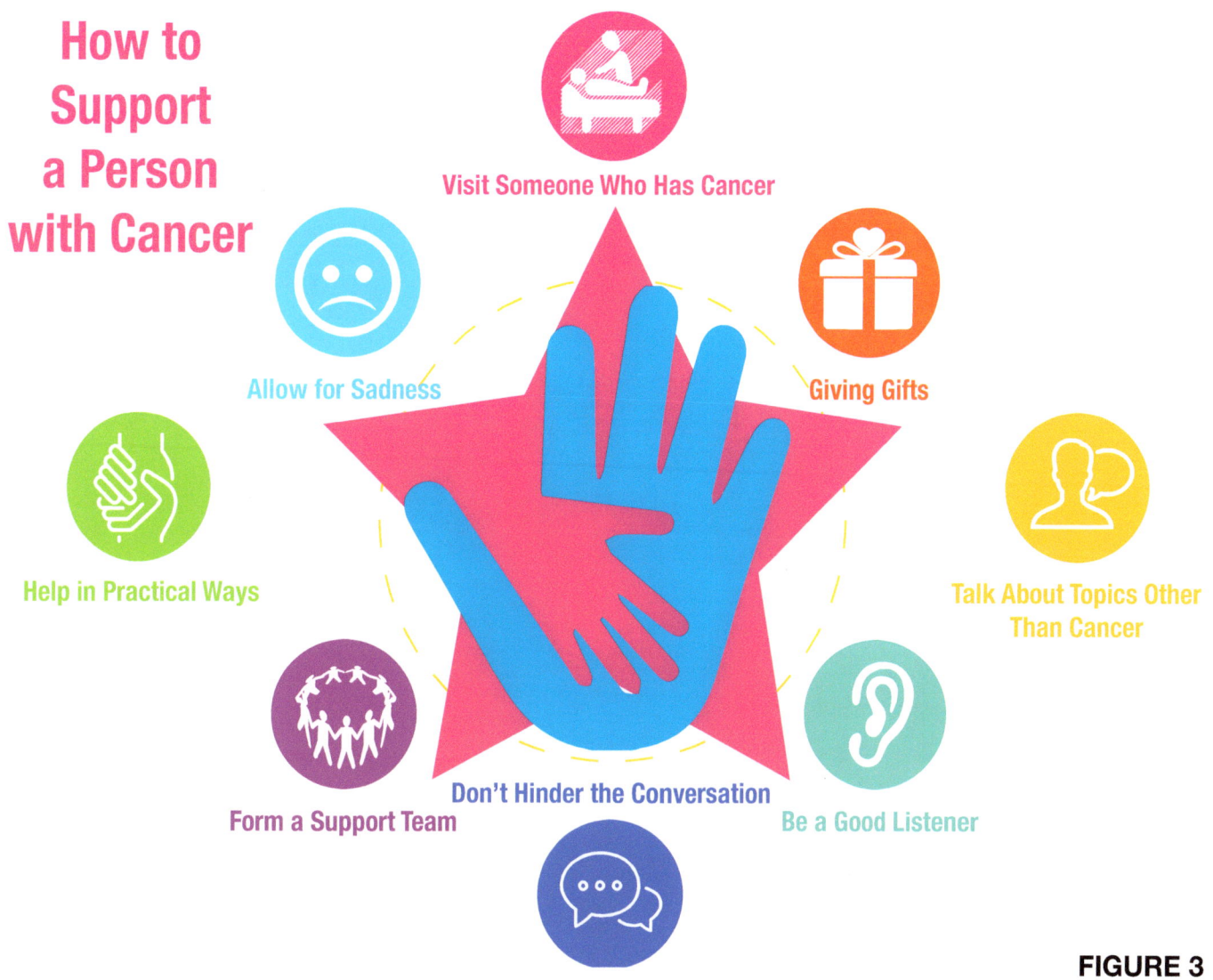

FIGURE 3

Mental Wellness - How to deal with Psychological Stress of Cancer

Mental wellness seems to be often overlooked as a part of the holistic treatment or care to any form of cancer.

Breast cancer may bring on a range of emotions that interfere with person's normal functioning. Here are a few useful tips for enhancing the psychological well-being of cancer fighter/survivor and a caregiver. Find out how to boost your self-esteem and confidence while fighting cancer or caring for someone who does.

✓ **Psychotherapy and Counseling**
Seeking professional psychotherapy is equally important for both cancer fighter/survivor and a caregiver since it can help them work together to understand the diagnosis, cope with the diagnosis and the challenges of treatment and respect each other's needs. You may seek individual, couple, family and/or group therapy and counseling. [4]

✓ **Spiritual Counseling**
Spiritual counseling for faith-based cancer fighters and their caregivers can be a vital part of a holistic treatment. Spiritual wellness may bring a sense of calm and peace to both fighter and caregiver and help them cope with the diagnosis and treatment.

✓ **Self-Help Skills**

EXERCISE mindful meditation. Mindfulness can help you focus on your feelings and thoughts and distract you from negative and destructive thoughts. Furthermore, mindful meditation can help you relax and change a viewpoint about your disease. It will strengthen you to focus on what you can change, not on what you can't change about your condition.

ESTABLISH a circle of support. Talk about your feelings. Reach out to family and friends, other cancer survivors a psychotherapist, or a spiritual leader.

MAKE healthy lifestyle choices. Pay attention to your needs for rest, nutrition, exercise and private time.

ENJOY a healthy humor. Humor has been used for years in medicine. Laughter therapy can lift your spirits and help you cope with negative feelings such as depression, fatigue, grief and low self-esteem. [5] For more information on laughter therapy, please go to https://www.cancercenter.com/treatments/laughter-therapy/

PRACTICE cancer affirmations. Cancer affirmations are positive and direct statements regarding the patient's condition and his/her ability to cope. The link between our mind and body has been given much more attention in recent decades. Mindfulness can help you make the positive changes in your body with positive thoughts.
To read more about positive affirmations for cancer fighters and survivors and their caregivers alike, please visit http://www.healthguidance.org/entry/11744/1/Cancer-Affirmations-Can-You-Really-Think-Yourself-Better.html

TRY coloring therapy. Different studies show that coloring pre-drawn Mandalas can help ease stress and anxiety symptoms and lead to relaxation of both mind and body. Coloring therapy has effects similar to mindful meditation – it helps you concentrate only on coloring task, and let go of negative thoughts. [6]
To learn more about coloring therapy benefits for cancer patients, go to https://www.tandfonline.com/doi/

For many people, seeking a professional psychotherapy and/or spiritual counseling is a vital part of their fight with cancer, whether it is coping with the diagnosis, treatment or recovery process. However, benefits of mental wellness and self-help are numerous. Self-care techniques such as humor, positive affirmations or coloring therapy can help you relieve stress, relax, and think positive while going through this important stage in your life. On the following pages, you will find a variety of mental wellness activities such as color comfort, poetry, challenging puzzles and sudoku, inspirational quotes, affirmations and intentions, humor, spirit animals, uplifting scriptures, and mindfulness meditations.

---

[1] National Cancer Institute, "Cancer Statistics", Last updated March 22nd 2017, https://www.cancer.gov/about-cancer/understanding/statistics

[2] Mayo Clinic Staff, "Breast Cancer", Mayo Clinic, 2018, https://www.mayoclinic.org/diseasesconditions/breast-cancer/symptoms-causes/syc-20352470

[3] Jim, Heather S.L., "History of Major Depressive Disorder Prospectively Predicts Worse Quality of Life in Women with Breast Cancer", US National Library of Medicine National Institutes of Health, 2013, https://www.ncbi.nlm.nih.gov/pmc/articles/PMC3424106/

[4] American Cancer Society, "Making Strides Against Breast Cancer", Cancer Survivors Network, 2018, https://secure.acsevents.org/site/SPageServer/?pagename=strides_msabc

[5] Cancer Treatment Centers of America, "Laughter Therapy", Cancer Treatment Centers of America, 2018, https://www.cancercenter.com/treatments/laughter-therapy/

[6] Eaton J., Tieber C., "The Effects of Coloring on Anxiety, Mood and Perseverance", Art Therapy, Journal of American Art Therapy Association, Published Online 22 February 2017, p. 42-46

Color Comfort

1

Color breathes life into everything and gives sensational beauty to the world around us. There are studies that show how important color is to our moods and how different colors can affect a person's demeanor or perception of something. Make your artwork a personal expression of yourself and the best it can be.

The mandala is a sacred circle. The word mandala comes from the ancient Sanskrit language and loosely means "circle" or "center." It's a simple geometric shape that has no beginning or end. Within its circular shape, the mandala is believed to have the power to promote relaxation, balance the body's energies, enhance your creativity, and support healing. Zentagles are beautiful repetitive patterns known as tangles that are believed to give focus and energy with satisifcation to the artists along with an increased sense of personal well-being.

Color for comfort by having fun with your mandala and zentagles coloring pages to your current mood. There are a variety of pencils, markers, pens, and crayons (watercolor, scented, gel, glazed/3-D, paint, pastels, & erasable) with a variety of tips shapes (fine, brush, bullet, chisel) and bases (water, oil, alcohol, & wax) to create your unique artwork! Relax, select your colors, plan your work and starting point; then, allow your mind to focus on coloring your mandala and zentagles!

See the Color Wheel to determine your choice of colors for your mandala and zentagles patterns in this section.

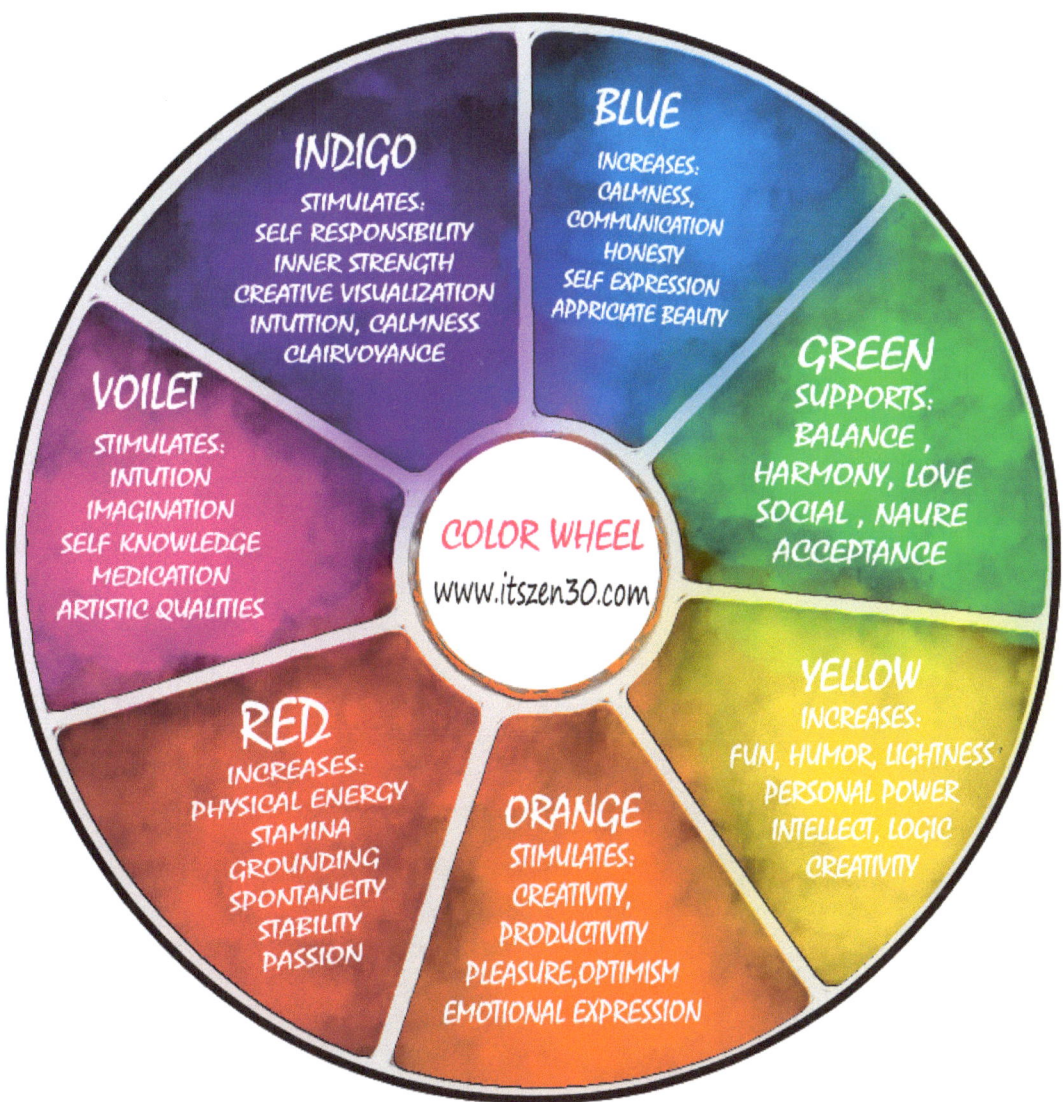

Permission to use the color was given by Augusto Herrera & Chantel Rodriguez of YOGART- COLOR THERAPY YOGA. Instagram: @itszen30 Email: now@itszen30.com

A gift to you from YOGART is free shipping on any single order of mood shades & all other items use code: '2020' to get 20% off (excludes discounted sets). www.itszen30.com

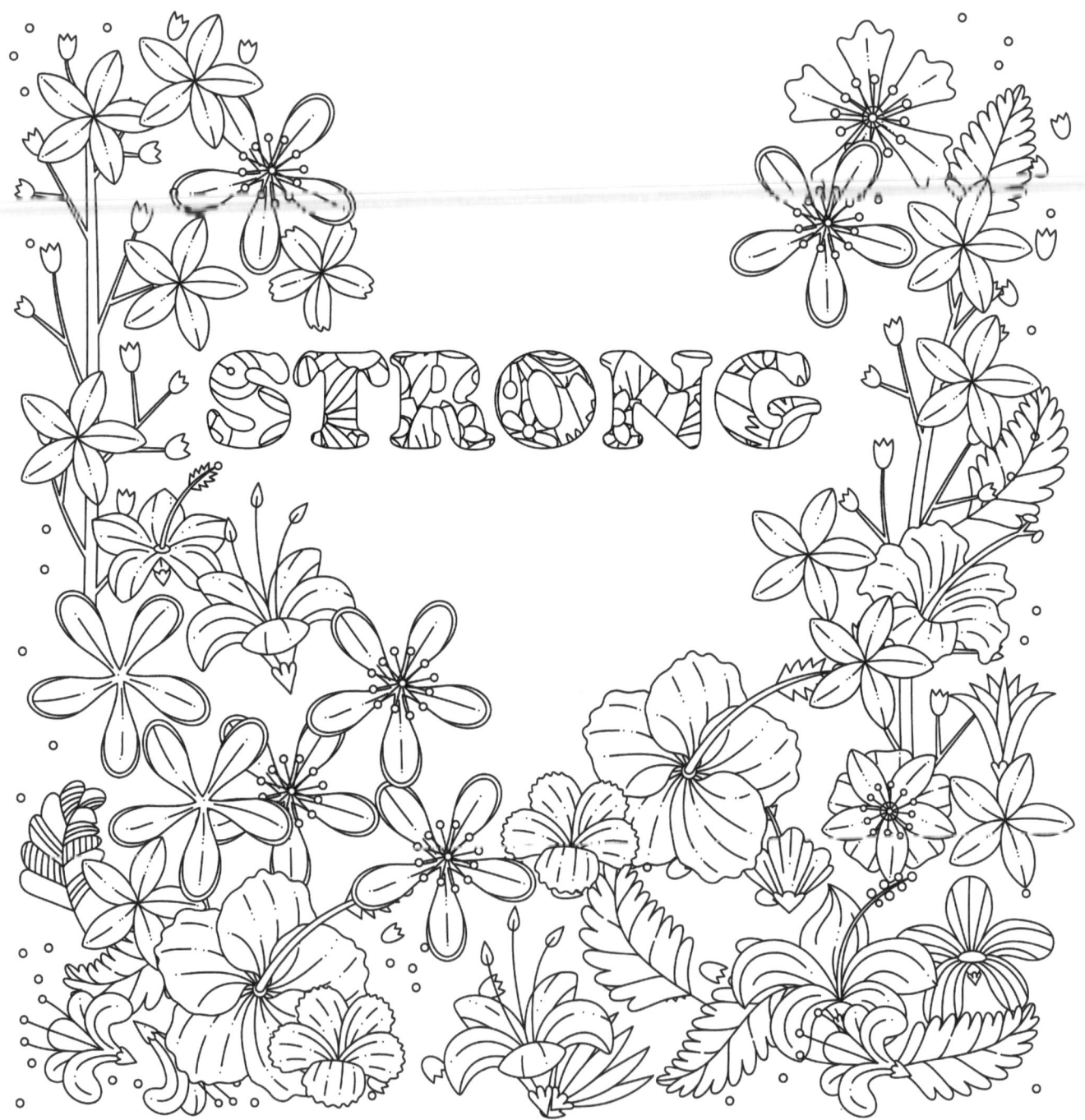

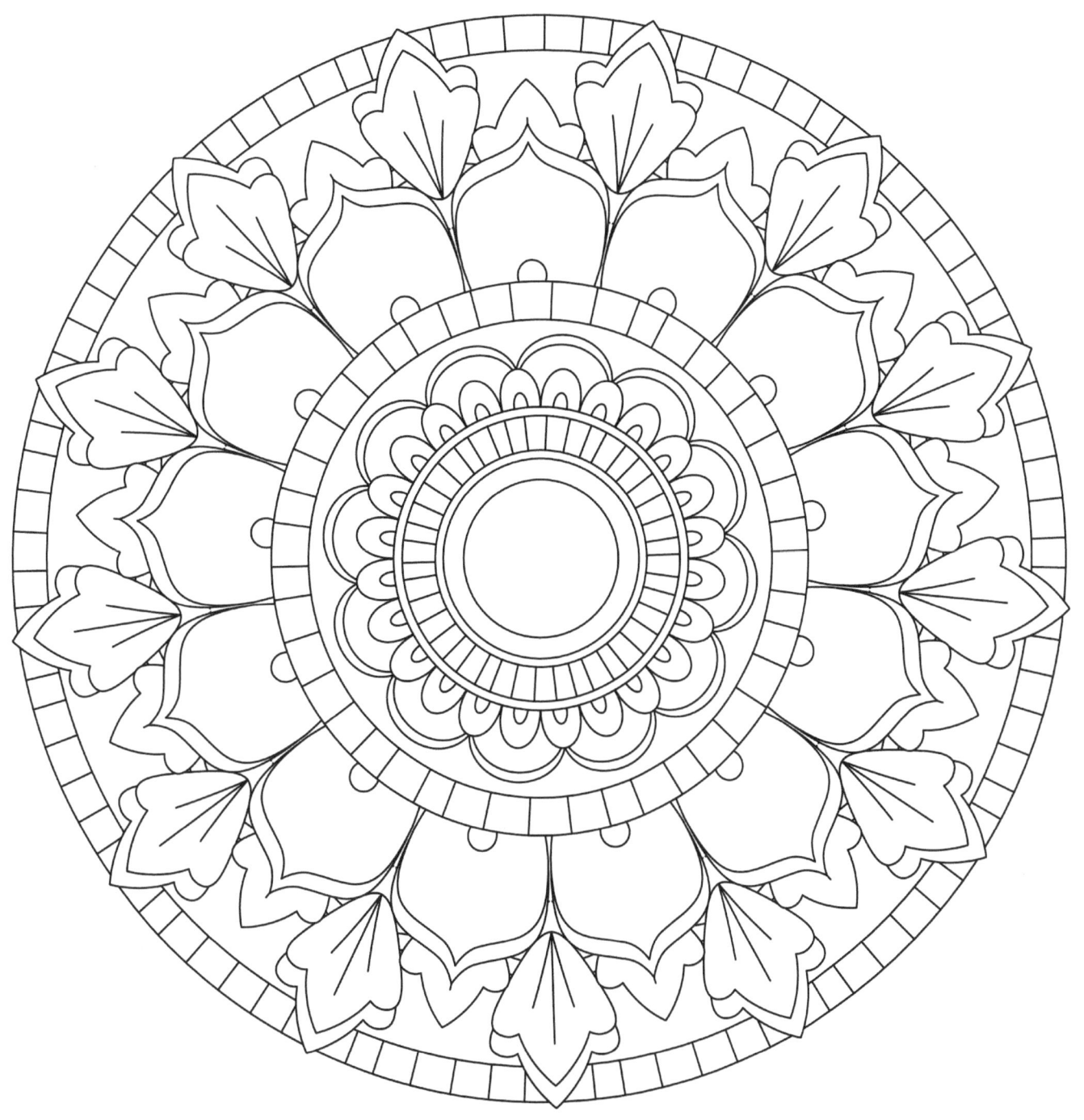

My artwork reflects my colorful mood(s). List words from the color wheel and/or your inner thoughts and feelings that symbolize your mood

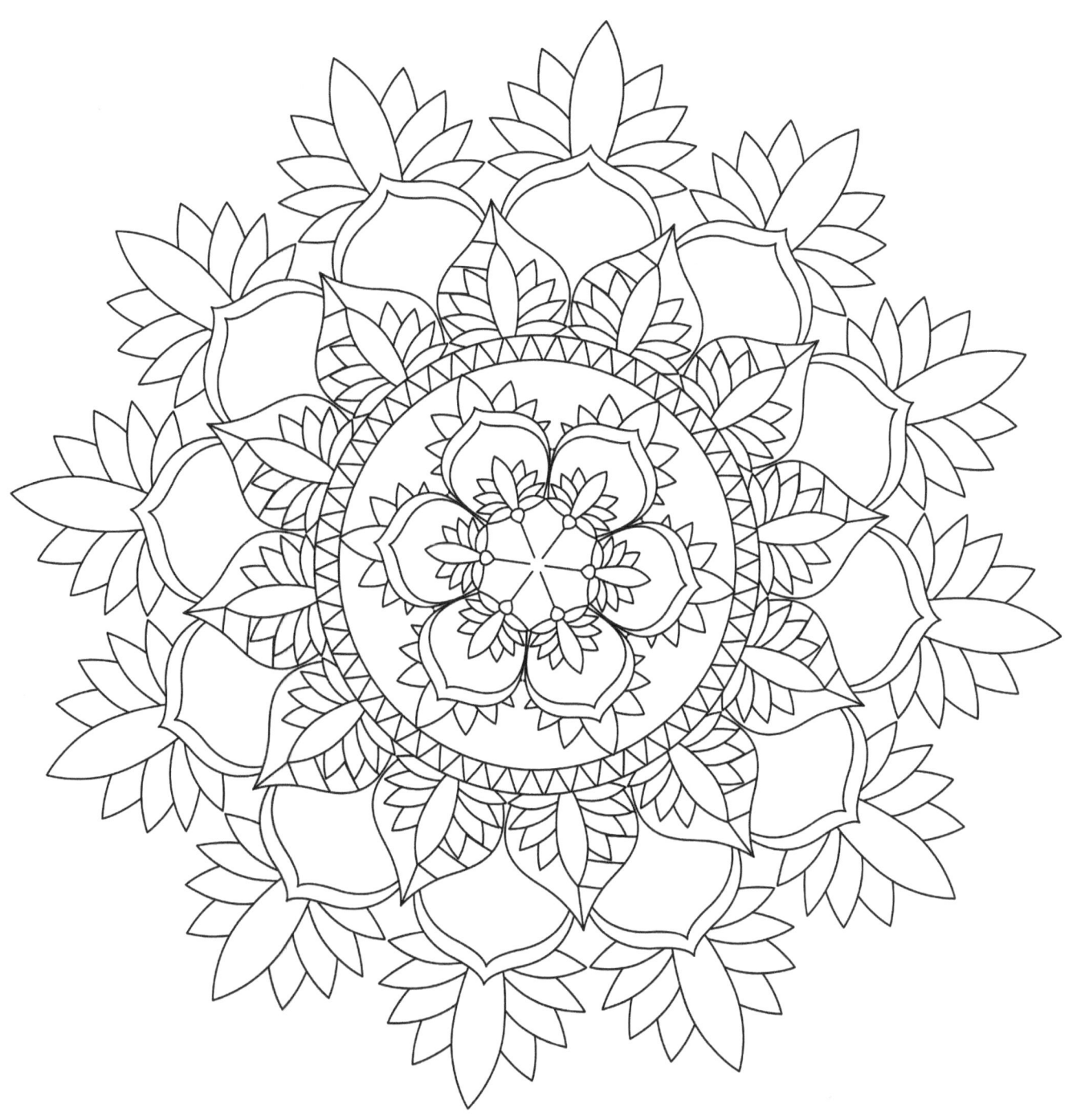

My artwork reflects my colorful mood(s).
List words from the color wheel and/or your inner thoughts and feelings that symbolize your mood

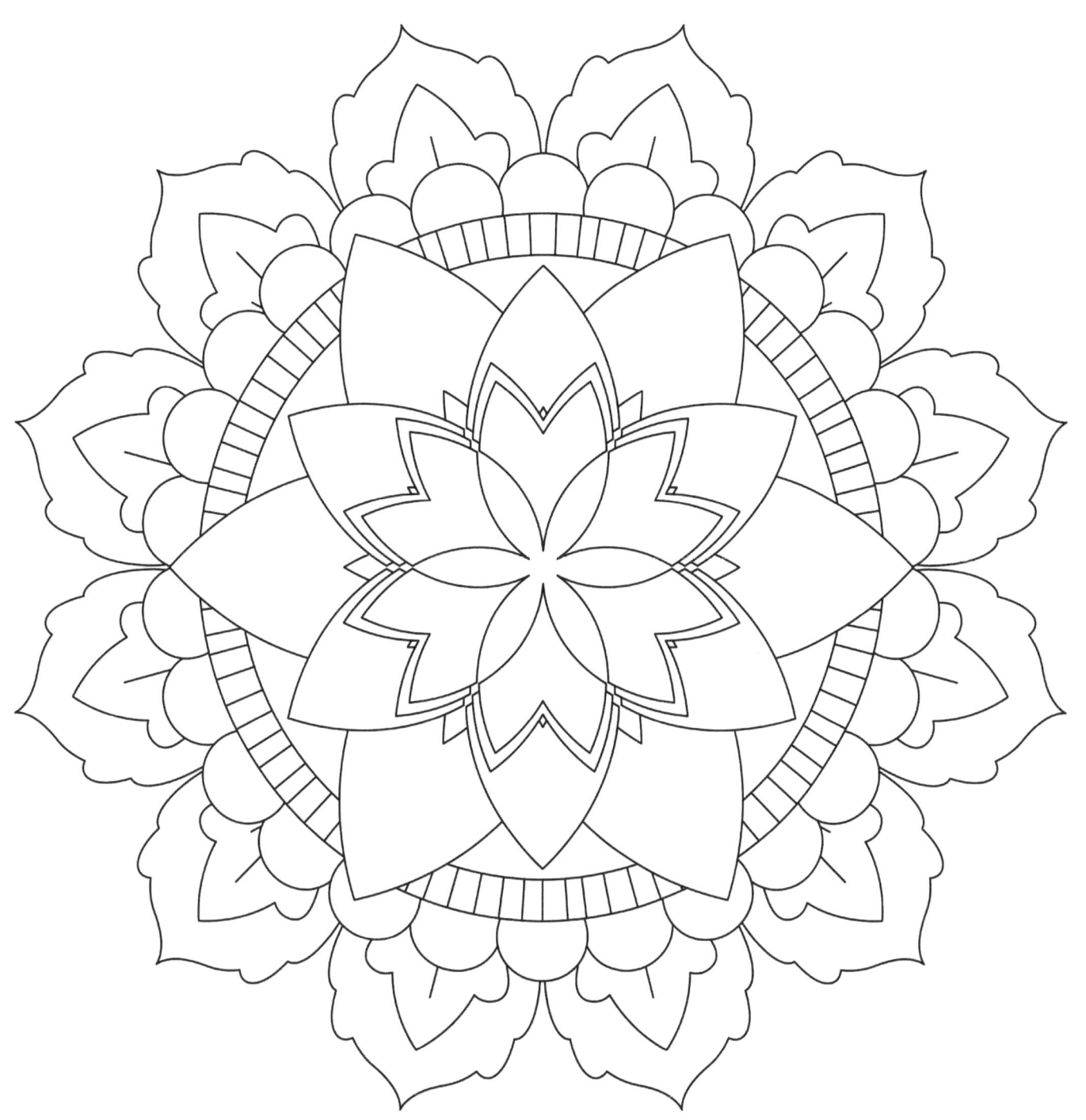

My artwork reflects my colorful mood(s).
List words from the color wheel and/or your inner thoughts and feelings that symbolize your mood

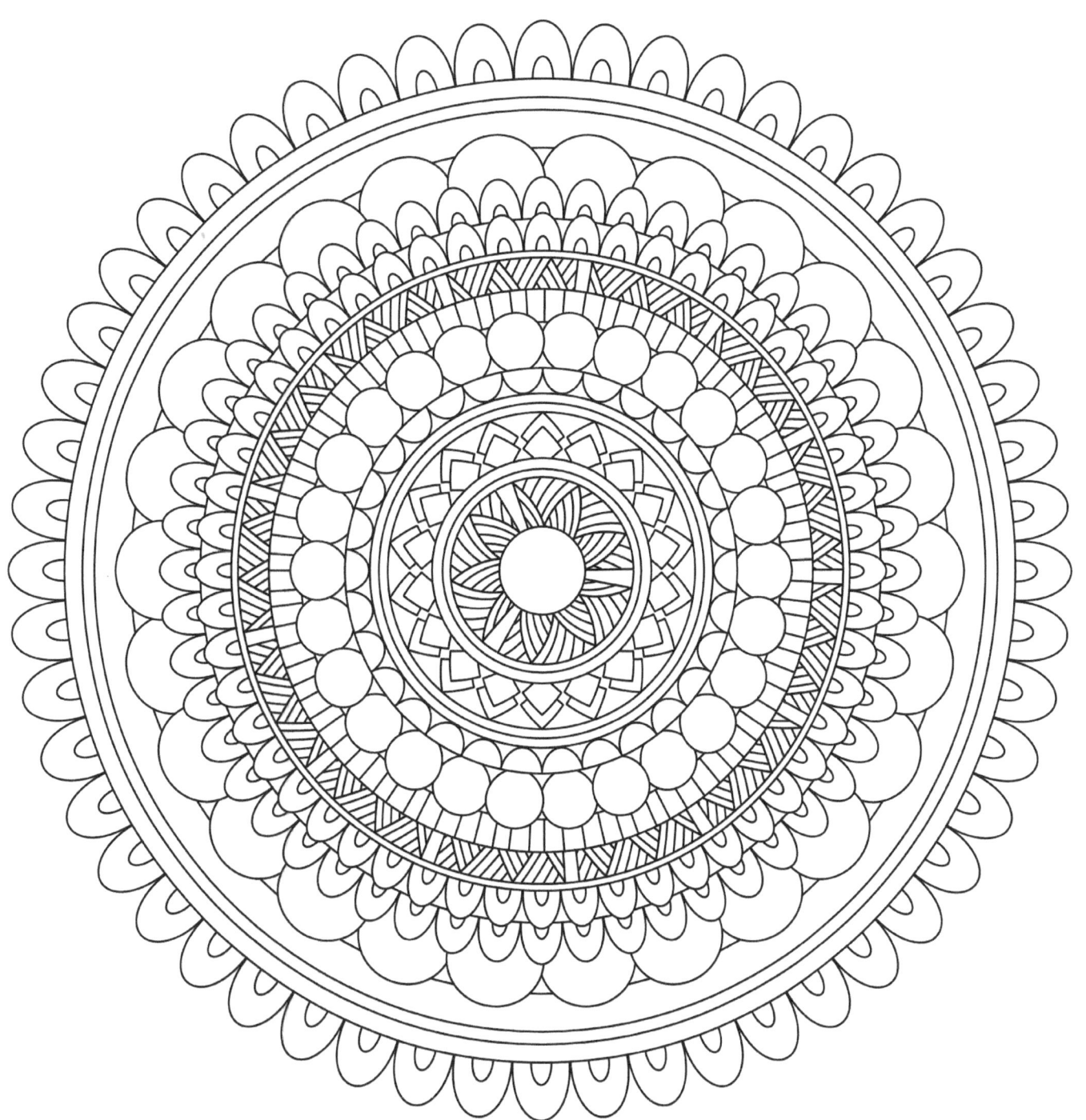

My artwork reflects my colorful mood(s). List words from the color wheel and/or your inner thoughts and feelings that symbolize your mood

_____

_____

_____

_____

_____

_____

_____

_____

_____

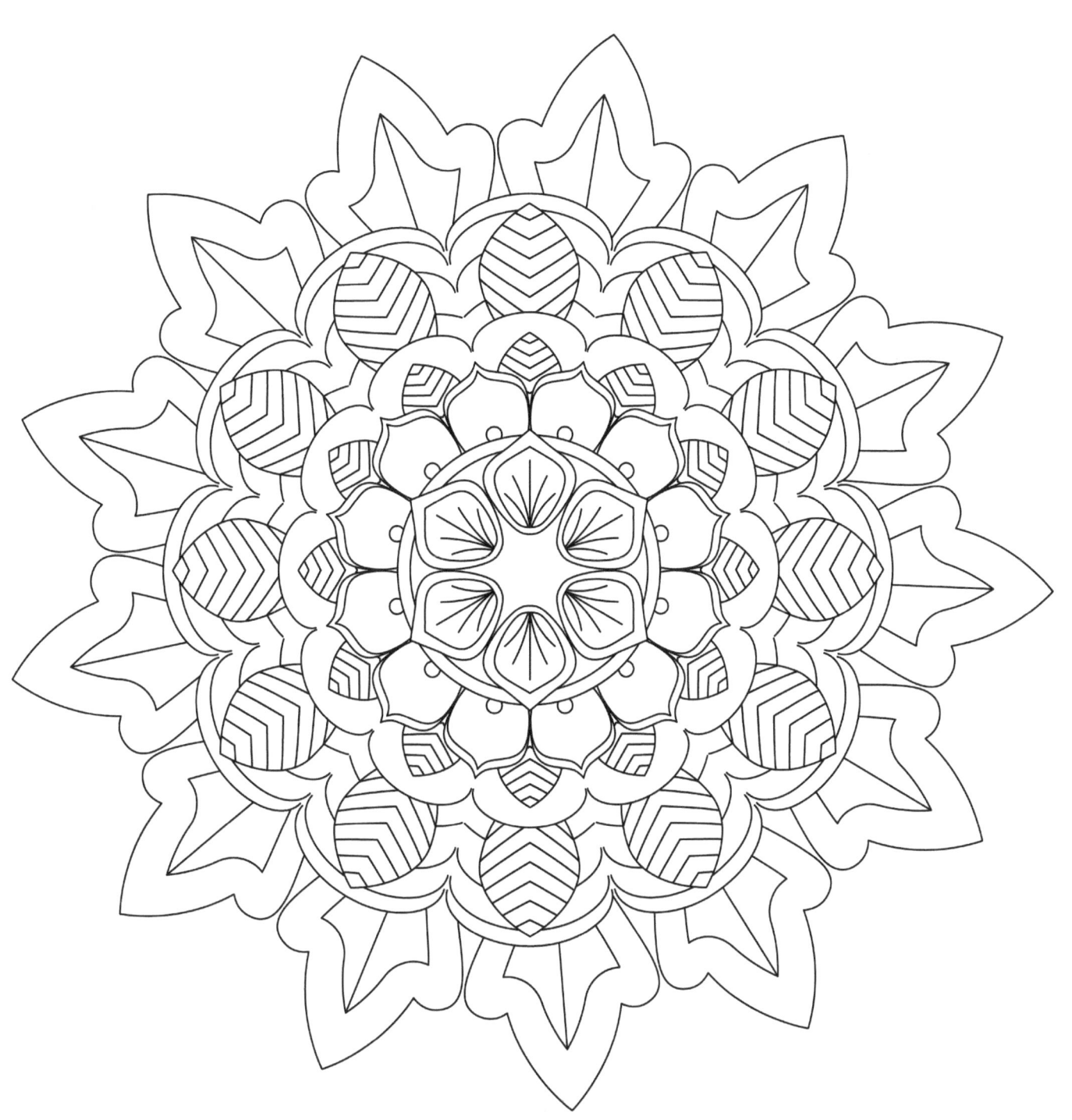

My artwork reflects my colorful mood(s).
List words from the color wheel and/or your inner thoughts and feelings that symbolize your mood

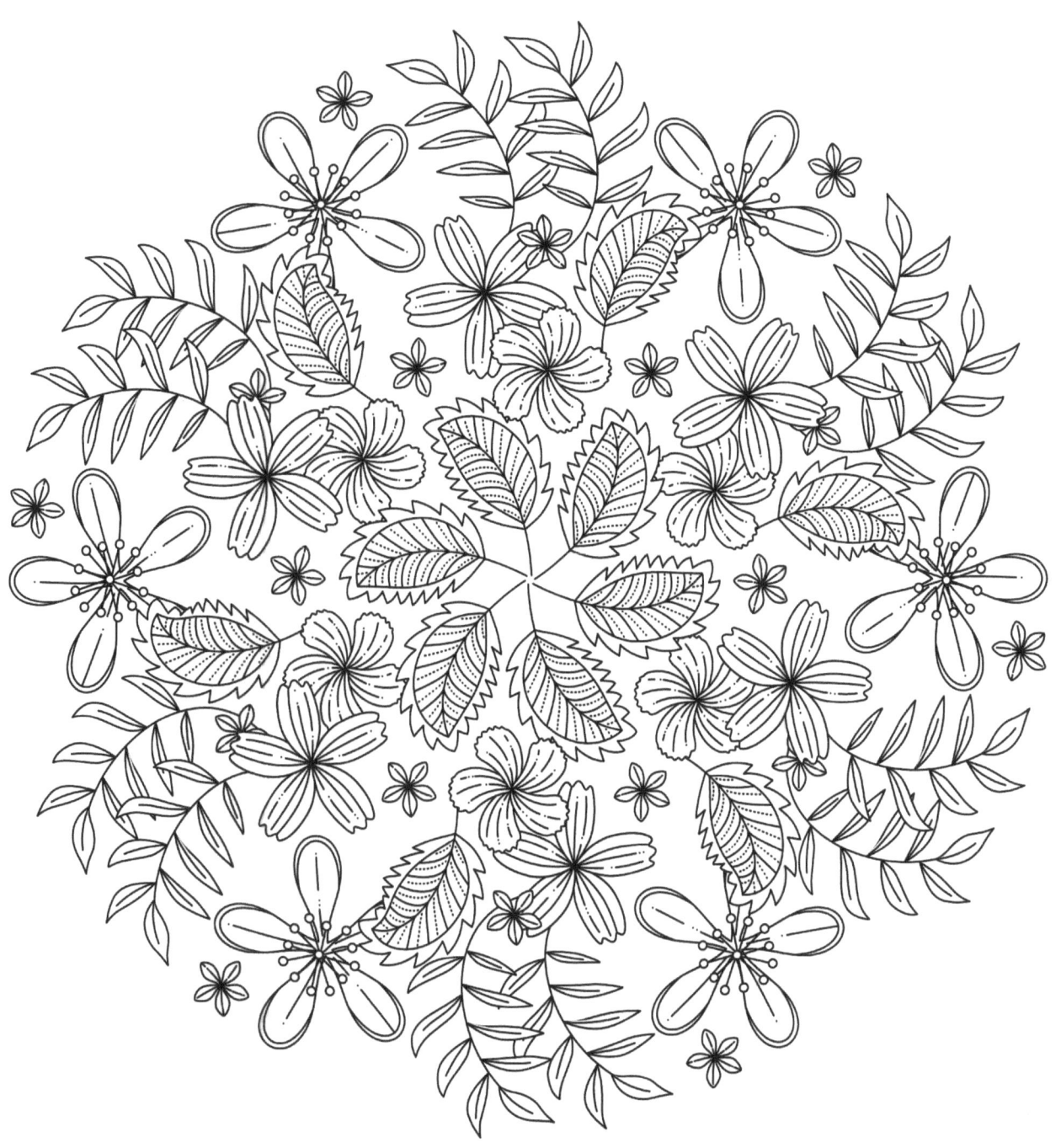

My artwork reflects my colorful mood(s). List words from the color wheel and/or your inner thoughts and feelings that symbolize your mood

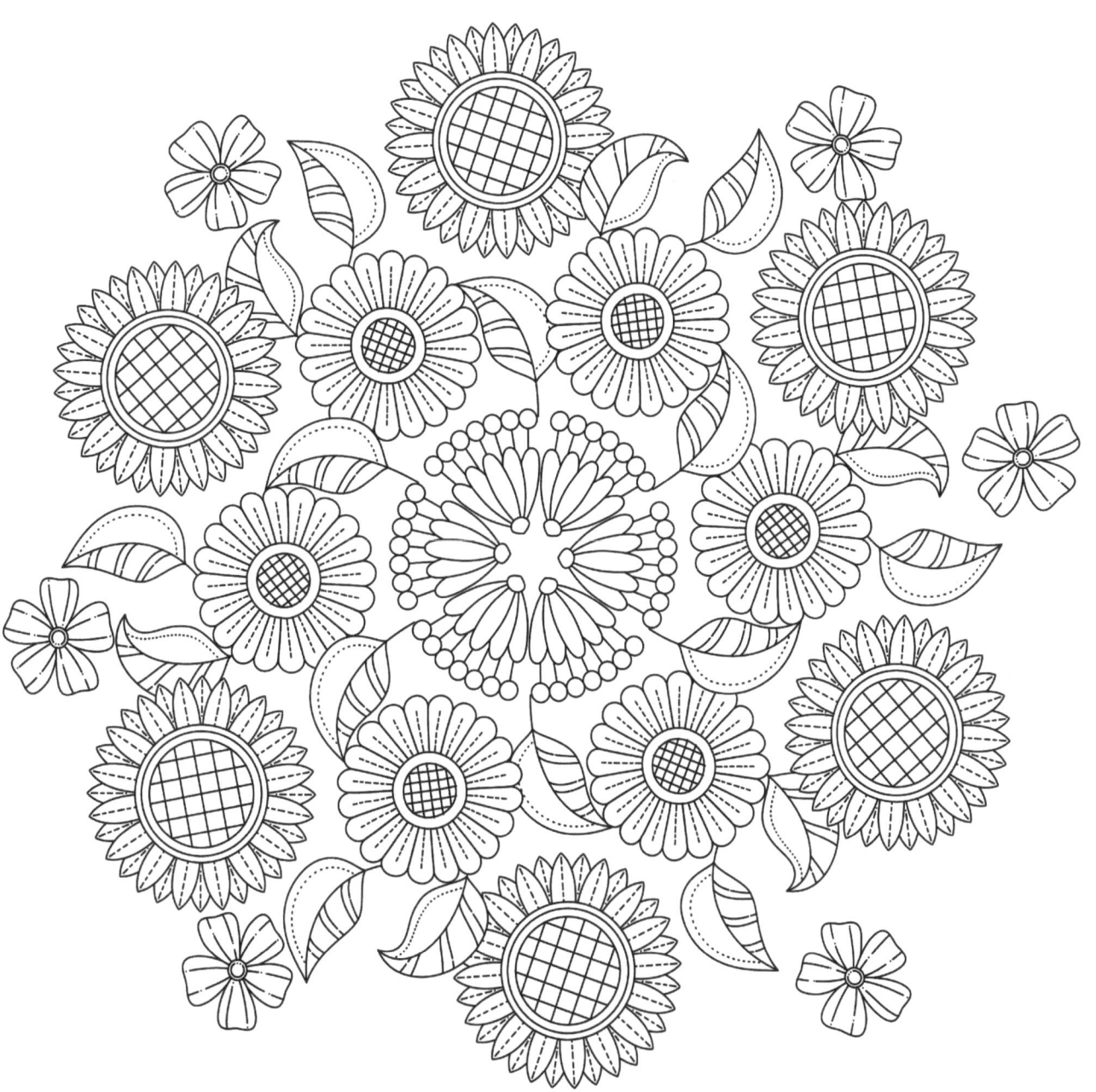

My artwork reflects my colorful mood (s). List words from the color wheel and/or your inner thoughts and feelings that symbolize your mood

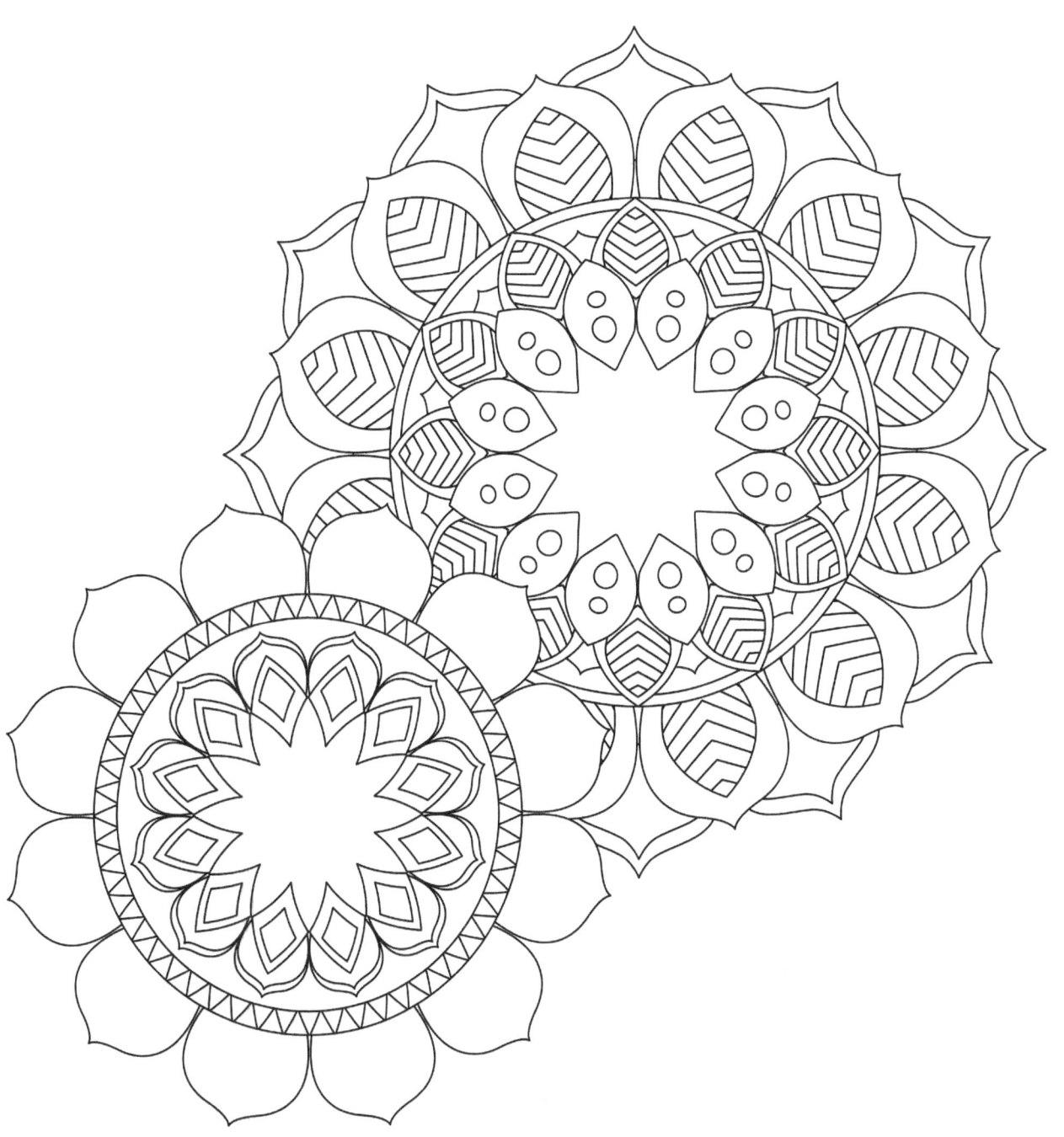

My artwork reflects my colorful mood (s).
List words from the color wheel and/or your inner thoughts and feelings that symbolize your mood

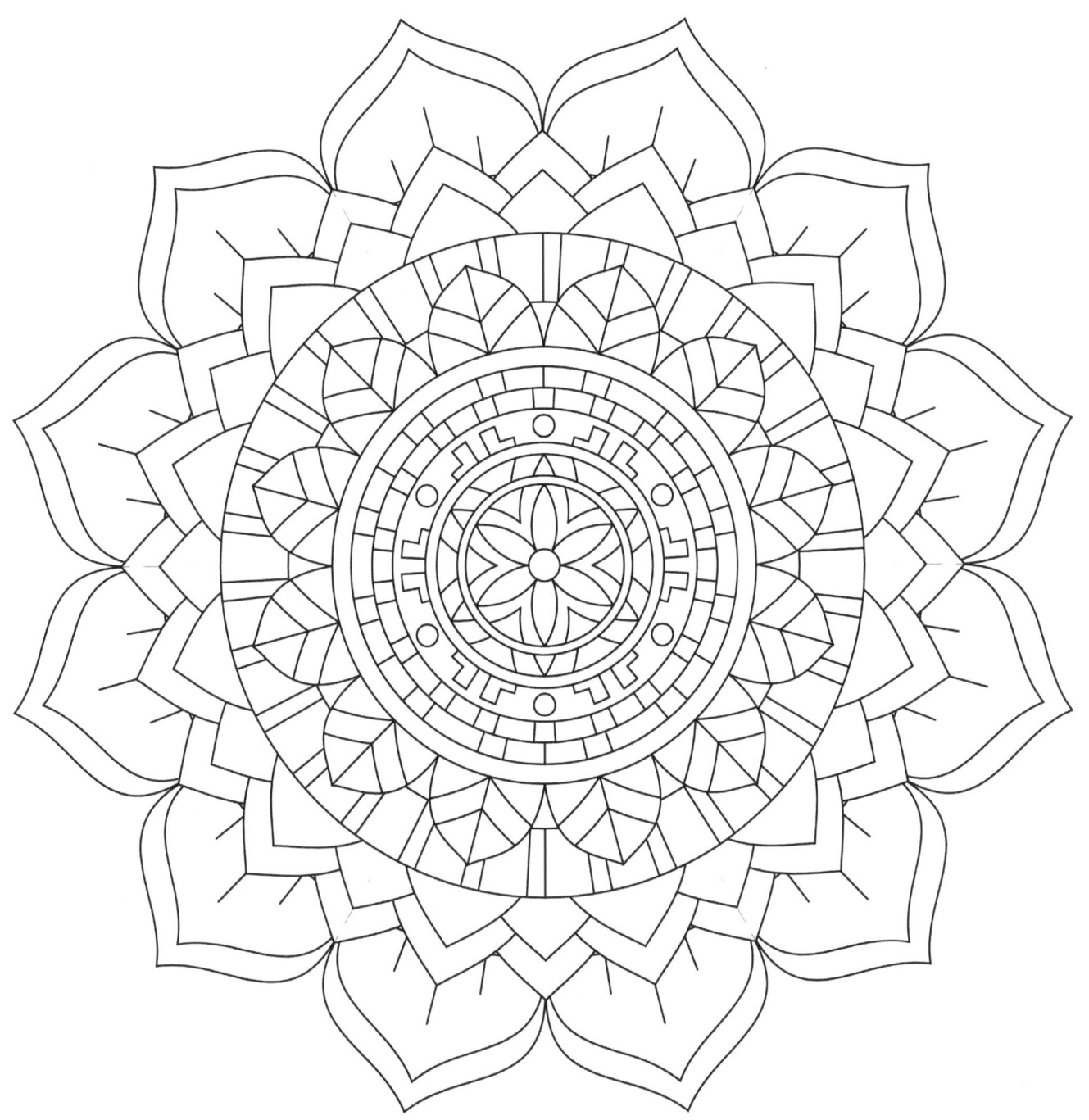

*My artwork reflects my colorful mood (s).
List words from the color wheel and/or your inner thoughts and feelings that symbolize your mood*

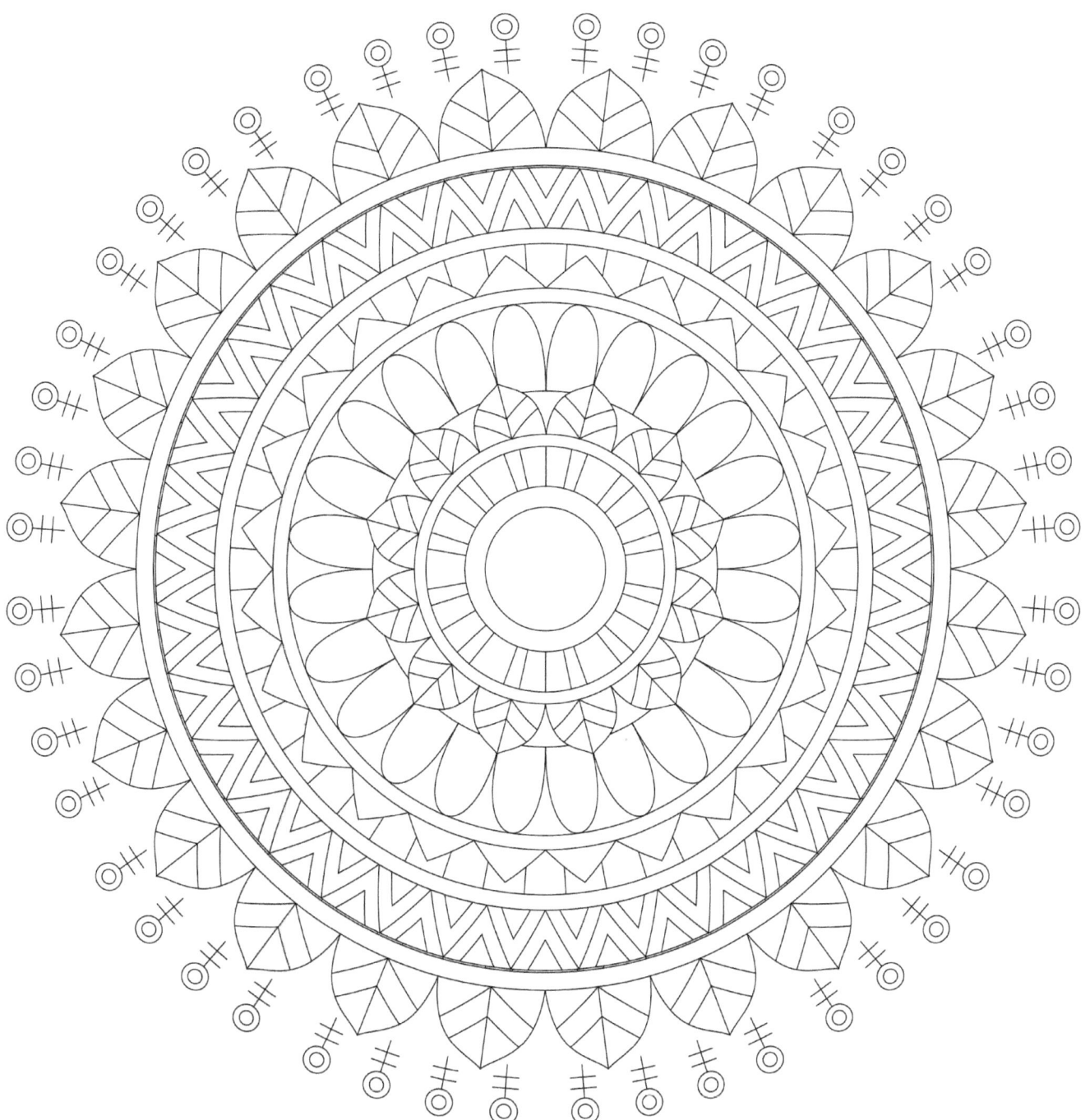

*My artwork reflects my colorful mood(s).
List words from the color wheel and/or your inner thoughts and feelings that symbolize your mood*

_____

_____

_____

_____

_____

_____

_____

_____

_____

_____

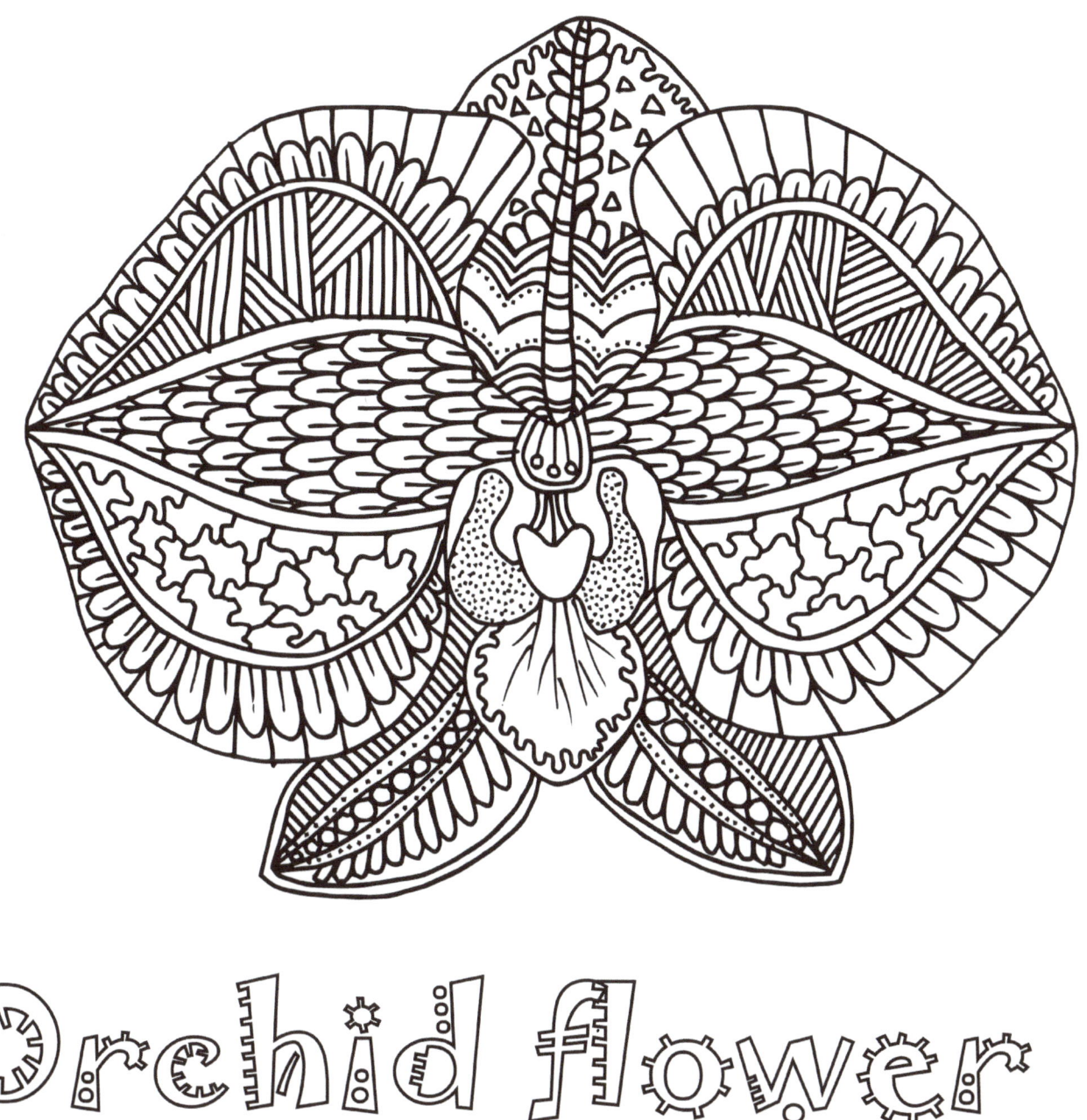

Orchid flower

Poetry
2

A Thought...a Word... a Visual Image... a Poem!

The poetry was written with a lot of love, faith, hope and visual thought for the breast cancer fighter, caregiver, and supporter of awareness. A single poem -- heart-rending, fearful, raging, beautiful, grotesque, even hilarious -- lets you know you are not alone in dealing with cancer. Poems have also been viewed as carriers of messages from the unconscious to the conscious mind. Wherever people gather to mark a moment, they speak from heart to heart, with poetry. These are lines to carry in our hearts, because they open us to beauty, a sense of self, healing, truth, and human connection, and all this in just a few words! The poems inspire hope to thrive and survive with cancer!

More THAN THEY SEE

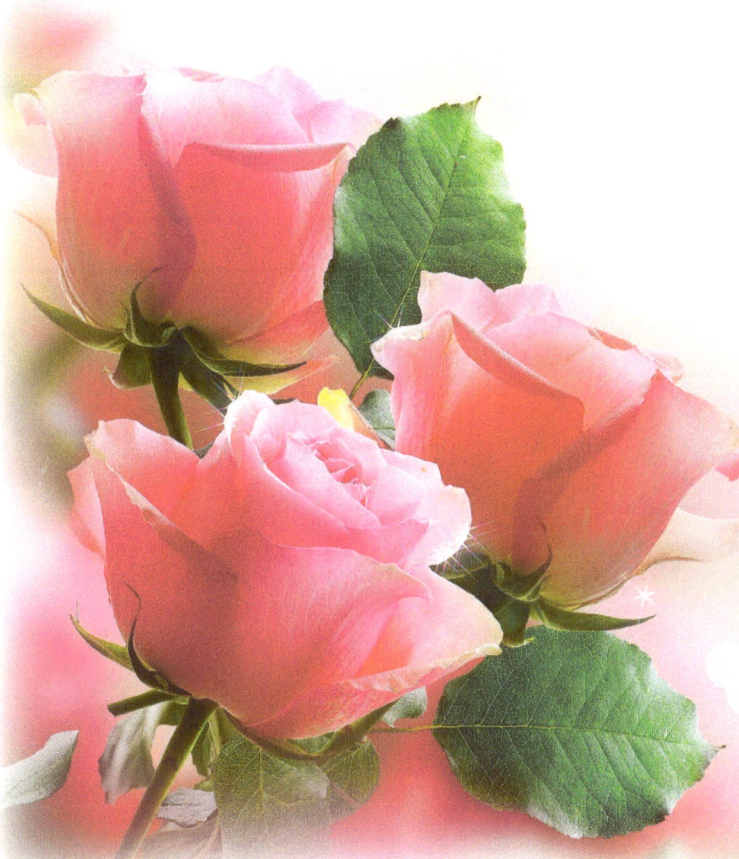

You are more than they see

You are a survivor
A conqueror and an encouragement
You make others see more of what they can become
In my eyes, you are perfect
You have done what most are afraid to do
You pushed yourself to get better
You stand before me right now the best version of yourself

You are more than they see
No one should ever tell you otherwise
You are unique and I love you
You are the one I look up to
Breast cancer couldn't pull you down
You continue to live your life
Show your strengths and share the happiness
A world without you is meaningless

You are more than they see
You have a story to tell
A life to live and a world to fill
Make the fight known to them
Make them see that this is not a joke
Your journey has just begun
And your path is paved clear
You are supposed to be a hero
I believe in you

You are more than they see
You are a mother, a father, a friend
You are a sister, a brother, a cousin to the end
You have to fight for us; you have to fight for you
They say you are more than they see

Do you know why?
Because you conquered the cancer
And now, you have a chance to educate on it too
I love you strong as you are
I know you feel it too

Strength WITHIN NUMBERS

Your dear loved one is fighting the battle of breast cancer
It is a battle meant to be won, and with you, it is a battle already won
Love is the most powerful force in the world
And your love for them is a fierce weapon to be reckoned with
You stand by their side, at the battlefront ready and waiting for what's next
Your support and strength drives them forward, it ignites their fire
As long as you are with them, they are sure to never tire
You look at them with pride and hope
The best is yet to come, and you both keep this in mind
As you brace yourselves with the pink ribbon tied across your arms
Your armor is a powerful source of hope, and an inner drive that's unmeasurable
You are strong
This battle may be long, but as long as you keep the flame of strength hot
Your breast cancer fighter will become stronger yet
Let love and support guide you both in this fierce battle
The sunrise is alive today with the knowledge of your prevail
The sky paints a story, one of a mighty warrior and their companions
The opponent is fierce, but this is of an inspiring ending, a grand and happy tale
The tale of two mighty warriors fighting with hope and love
The battle of breast cancer is far from over, we are all cheering you on
With that pink ribbon and radiant belief
You serve as a symbol for perseverance and strength, within numbers
Your loved one looks to you for guidance
All you need to give is your undying support
Since there is infinite might within numbers

TO BE *Strong*

To just breathe, to allow your lungs to expand
To continue this steady act of simply breathing when things seem impossible
You don't know that this, this is to be strong
Little do you know, you're steadily fanning your inner flame
With each breath
The fire within your heart sizzles louder, serving as a beacon to hope
To be strong when this illness blows its harsh winds
You might even see the strength as a twinkle in your eye
Your eyes reveal the fire of burning strength
Nothing could ever stomp out your flame
You are strong and beautiful
The winds only serve to fan your flames, to make you even stronger
Never doubt yourself, because to be strong
The hardships you may face can seem so long
Just know that, this battle is far from over
Recognize the breath within your magnificent lungs
Simply this, is to be strong
There is infinite beauty inside of your soul
You may see the present as a steep hill
But since you possess an inner fire
To win such a battle
You will

Puzzles
3

A puzzle is a great way to pass idle or spare moments by indulging in word searches, crossword puzzles, word scramble, or sudoku. There are puzzles related to breast cancer awareness and just for fun in this section! The puzzles should engage your mind and keep you entertained, especially if you love a brain challenge to get a vigorous mental workout while learning useful tips related to breast cancer and just having fun! Activate your brain cells and grab a pencil -solve the puzzles for fun or to learn a tip or two!

NOTE: The sudoku puzzles answers are in the appendix of the book.

BREAST CANCER

Fill in the squares with the words from the right.
Then find out what the message is below.

believe
cherish
courage
cure
determined
faith
hope
love
peace
strength

being ⬛ ⬛ ⬛ ⬛ *is still beautiful*

Answer: Bald

Activities to Pass Time

The crossword puzzle is in a shape of a heart to symbolize the love of life and how you can love yourself and life by keeping busy with activities. Be creative and use various color pens or pencils to find the activities in the word list that can help pass time and relieve stress daily!

```
            F X D           T L O
          Y O G A X       S L E E P
        C R O C H E T   W E E I V O M
        A W N O I T A C A V H C A E B
        H W G A R D E N I N G G S H K
        J G S N O I T A T I D E M R R
        C O L O R I N G F I S H I N G
          F A M I L Y T I M E S L Y
          W C B P C A R D G A M E V
            P I A U D I O B O O K
              I S T A L K I N G
                C U H G U A L
                  N M N Y S
                    I R B
                      C
```

WORD LIST:

AUDIO BOOK	FAMILY TIME	MOVIE	TALKING
BEACH VACATION	FISHING	MUSIC	YOGA
CARD GAME	GARDENING	PICNIC	
COLORING	LAUGH	SLEEP	
CROCHET	MEDITATIONS	SMILE	

SUDOKU PUZZLES

8	7	9	6		4			
4					3			
		6	9		8		7	4
	4	3	1			7	8	
			4				3	
			7	3		4		6
			2	6		1		7
2		1	8		7		6	
	6	7			1			2

3					1		8	2
	7	6	3	8		1		
							6	4
8	6	2		1	7		4	3
	5	9		2		6		
4								
7		5	1		9	4	2	
6	2			4	5			1
			2		8	5		

4	6			7			9	2
1	9	2		5	8			7
		7		2			4	1
	3				7		1	
	1	9					6	
	7	4					8	9
6		3			1	9	5	8
	5						4	6
				6	9			3

	3	9	1			4		2
		6					1	5
					5			9
1	7	2		8	6	5	9	
8	6	4		9	2			3
9	5	3						8
	4		2	7		9		
				5	8			7
		5			1	8		

54

Puzzle 1

4			1					
2	8			5	3			1
		7	2				3	6
	4	8	9	2	6	3	1	
3	5	9		1				
6	2			4		7	8	
	7				8			
	9	3		7	2	6		
		4	5			2		

Puzzle 2

9		3			8		1	
7				9				8
8	1			7			2	3
			8	3	4			2
				5			1	8
				7			3	9
6		4				3		
2	9		6		3	8	4	
3	8			4	7			

			7	8			2	1
				3	9	5		6
	2		9	5		8		
		5						
4	3	2	1	8				5
8		6			4			2
2	6	4	7	1	9	5	8	
				2		1	4	9
1			4	3	5			

	3		6	9	4	1		7
	9		3	1			6	
	6	1			2		8	3
	5	8	2	3		7	4	
	7			8	6		5	2
				4				
				5	1			
3	4	2				5	9	
5		9						

Puzzle 1

	5	8			2		3	7
		2		4		6		1
		6	1	8	7	5	9	2
	6		2					
	7			6	1	2		
	8	1			4			
8				3			1	
5			7					4
		7	4	2	8			

Puzzle 2

		2	8	4				
			5		7	6		
7					2	1	4	8
		1		5	3			4
	2		4	8	6	7		
	4		1					
4	7	6		1			8	9
5	1	9					7	3
	3	8	9		4			

Healthy Eating: Fruits & Vegetables

Good nutrition is to key to any persons healthy eating plan. Have fun and discover foods that are nutritional and tasty!

Across

2 Round, glossy red, typically eaten with salad
4 Round, juicy yellow flesh, sweet, hard pit in the middle
8 Melon like, smooth green skin, red pulp, watery juice
9 Long, pointed, orange root
11 A hard shell dry fruit or seed, can be plain or salted
12 Round, purple, green, red, or black, grows in clusters on a grapevine
14 Green, round, seed-pod vegetable
15 Green, curled or wrinkled leaves, cabbage like plant

Down

1 Thick green or purple leaves, globular head
3 Long, pale green, juicy stems with small shoots at one end
5 Green or purplish flower buds, similar to cauliflower
6 Small, pulpy, edible fruit, multiple seeds and colors
7 Round, juicy, citrus fruit
10 Round, white, may cause you to tear when preparing
13 Round, yellow, red, or green skin, crisp flesh, good for making cider

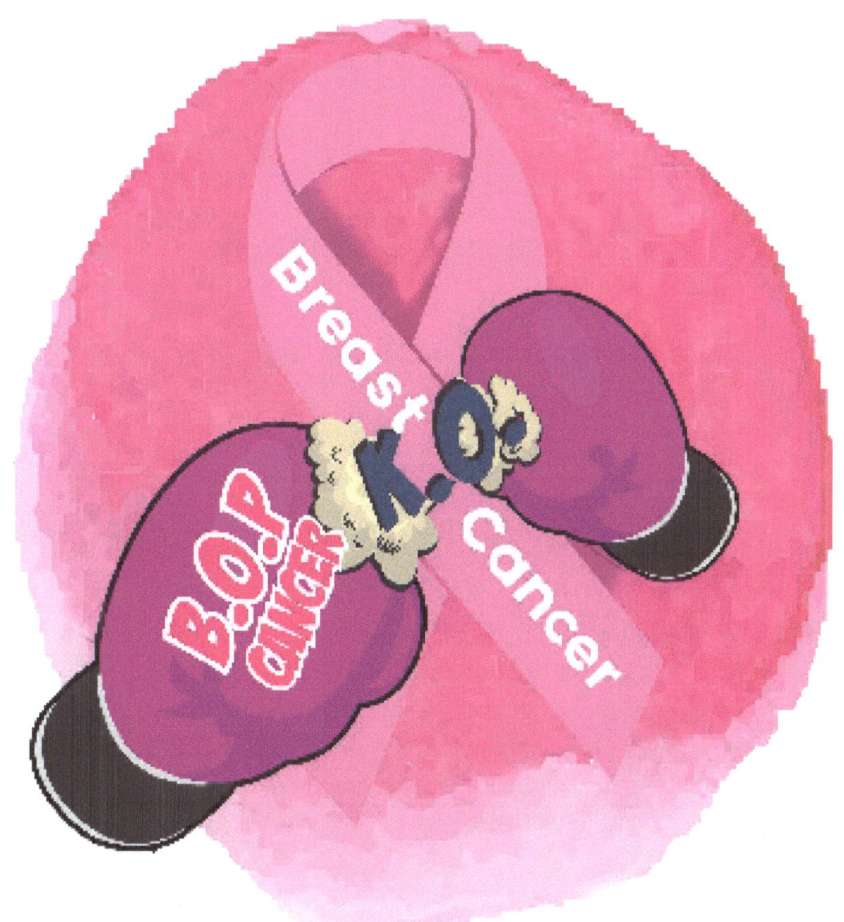

A state of well-being in your mind when you realize your own abilities to cope with life stressors_____.

Answer: Mental Wellness

Affirmations, Intentions & Inspirational Quotes

4

Words are believed to heal your heart and life. Some of the thoughts we think and words we say can give us hope for the future. It is helpful to use intentions and affirmations to release negative or painful thoughts to allow for more loving and compassionate thoughts. The Intention is a conscious reminder to all aspects of your being of what it is you want out of your life experience. Inspirational quotes are mental or emotional motivation intended to convey inspiration for your life. Affirmations are sentences aimed to affect the conscious and the subconscious mind, automatically and involuntarily, bringing up related mental images into the mind, which could inspire, energize and motivate you.

Uplift your outlook with a Total Knock Out (T.K.O.) of negative thoughts about cancer. Enjoy reading, saying in your mind or out loud the affirmations, intentions, or inspirational quotes in this section daily to uplift your spirits and positive mindset on living life! If you like, use the worksheet in this section to create your own Intentions and Affirmations!

FIGHTERS

Affirmation & Intentions

1 **My illness does not control me, it does not change me or make me less then I am.**
- I intend that I am separate from the illness.
- I intend that my identity, personality and all that I am has nothing to do with the illness.
- I intend that I know my worth and hold my value to the highest of standards.

2 **Illness will not cause me to change or rule me with fear.**
- I intend that I am fearless.
- I intend that I am courageous and strong.
- I intend that fear has no power over me.

3 **My body is strong, beautiful, and amazing.**
- I intend that I know the strength and beauty of my body.
- I intend that I never forget how amazing and extraordinarily capable my body is of healing itself.

4 **I trust my body to heal itself and remain strong, to always be beautiful, and to stay amazing.**
- I intend that I always trust in my body's abilities to heal itself.
- I intend that I can always see my beauty.
- I intend that I can always see the qualities and abilities within me that make me amazing.

5 **Cancer does not have power over me.**
- I intend that cancer have no power over me.

6 **I have the power to defeat it.**
- I intend that I have all the power within me to defeat cancer.

7 **I will not allow cancer to control me or my actions.**
- I intend that cancer has no control over me, my actions, thoughts or abilities.

8 **I inhale healthy air and exhale all that causes illness and pain.**
- I intend that vibrant, healing energy be inhaled and all that causes illness and pain be exhaled with each breath I take.

9 **I release all that damages my health and my body.**
- I intend that all damaging energies in my life be released and dispersed into the universe to do no more harm to me, my body, mind or soul.
- I intend that all energies in my life be healing energies that lift me up and give me strength.

10 **Cancer cannot take away who you are, but it can make you aware of your strength.**
- I intend that there are positive outcomes in all things.

11 **My body has the strength to conquer all it encounters.**
- I intend that my body has all of the strength it needs to conquer all it encounters.

12 **I can conquer all illness.**
- I intend that I conquer all things in my path.

13 **Illness can not conquer me.**
- I intend that nothing can conquer me.

14 **Cancer is not welcome in my body.**
- I intend that all cancer be dispelled from my body.

15 **I release all that is not welcome in my body and in my life.**
- I intend that I release all that no longer serves me from my body and from my life.

CAREGIVERS

Affirmation & Intentions

1. I am strong enough to do anything.
- I intend that I have the strength to conquer anything.

2. I can provide love and care for others and myself.
- I intend that I have the abilities to care for myself and others.
- I intend that I have enough love for myself and others.
- I intend that I have the time to care for myself.

3. My love and support is enough.
- I intend that whatever I have to give is enough.
- I intend that I know I am enough.

4. My best is enough, and I will get through this to what's next.
- I intend that I am doing my best.
- I intend that I will get through this with strength and grace.
- I intend that this is temporary.

5. When people stand together against cancer the beauty of being human can be seen.
- I intend that people stand together against all things.
- I intend that we all can see the beauty in one another.
- I intend that everyone know the beauty within themselves and one another simply for being human.

To do...

Now that you have read or spoken out loud the affirmations and intentions. Take a moment to complete the exercise on the following pages to customize your experience to your own thoughts of affirmations, intentions, and thankfulness.

Today's Date_____

Today I *intend* **that I** *feel*

Today I *intend* **that**

Today I am *thankful* **for**

Today's *affirmation*

Name 4 things you're *thankful* for in your personal life:

Name 4 things that happened this week to be *thankful* for:

Name 4 things you're *thankful* for in your professional life:

Name 4 skills you're *thankful* for:

Name 4 people you're *thankful* for in your life:

Name 4 personality traits you're *thankful* for:

Name 4 people in the world you're *thankful* for:

Name 4 physical aspects you're *thankful* for:

Name 4 subjects you're *thankful* for:

Name 4 modes of entertain you're *thankful* for:

INSPIRATIONAL
Quotes & Intentions

1. Cancer happens, people triumph.
- I intend that I remember this is not uncommon and people often triumph.
- I intend that I remember people beat this every day.

2. Breast cancer is everyone's struggle to be overcome together.
- I intend that everyone band together, to ease struggle and overcome.

3. Life is full of beauty but also intense challenges that must be faced.
- I intend that life is beautiful. Challenges and all.

4. Cancer cannot take away who you are, but it can make you aware of your strength.
- I intend there are positive outcomes in all things.

5. When people stand together against cancer the beauty of being human can be seen.
- I intend that people stand together against all things.
- I intend that we all can see the beauty in one another.
- I intend that everyone know the beauty within themselves and one another simply for being human.

HUMOR
5

A good belly laugh comes packed with many healthy psychological benefits. It releases endorphins, which are the feel-good chemicals in our brain that reduce pain and boost mood. Laughter makes us happy, offers a welcome distraction, and it's seriously fun. It can also be soothing, especially for those with lots of stress and worry on their minds. Some cancer patients find that laughing out loud, especially in the company of friends and family is helpful to relieve stress.
In this section, I invite Fighters and Caregivers to laugh, not to be forced into it. If you can, allow yourself to see the funny, it may lead to a new perspective as you find the humor in the comics or jokes. This section intends to take what can be a challenging experience and turn it into something humorous. May you see the humor in the comics and jokes with an open mind to LOL (laugh out loud)!

Disclaimer: The jokes are written in a general manner and are not intended to offend anyone who has, had, or caregivers to anyone with cancer. The reading of this section is voluntary, if you do not like this section, please skip reading this section.

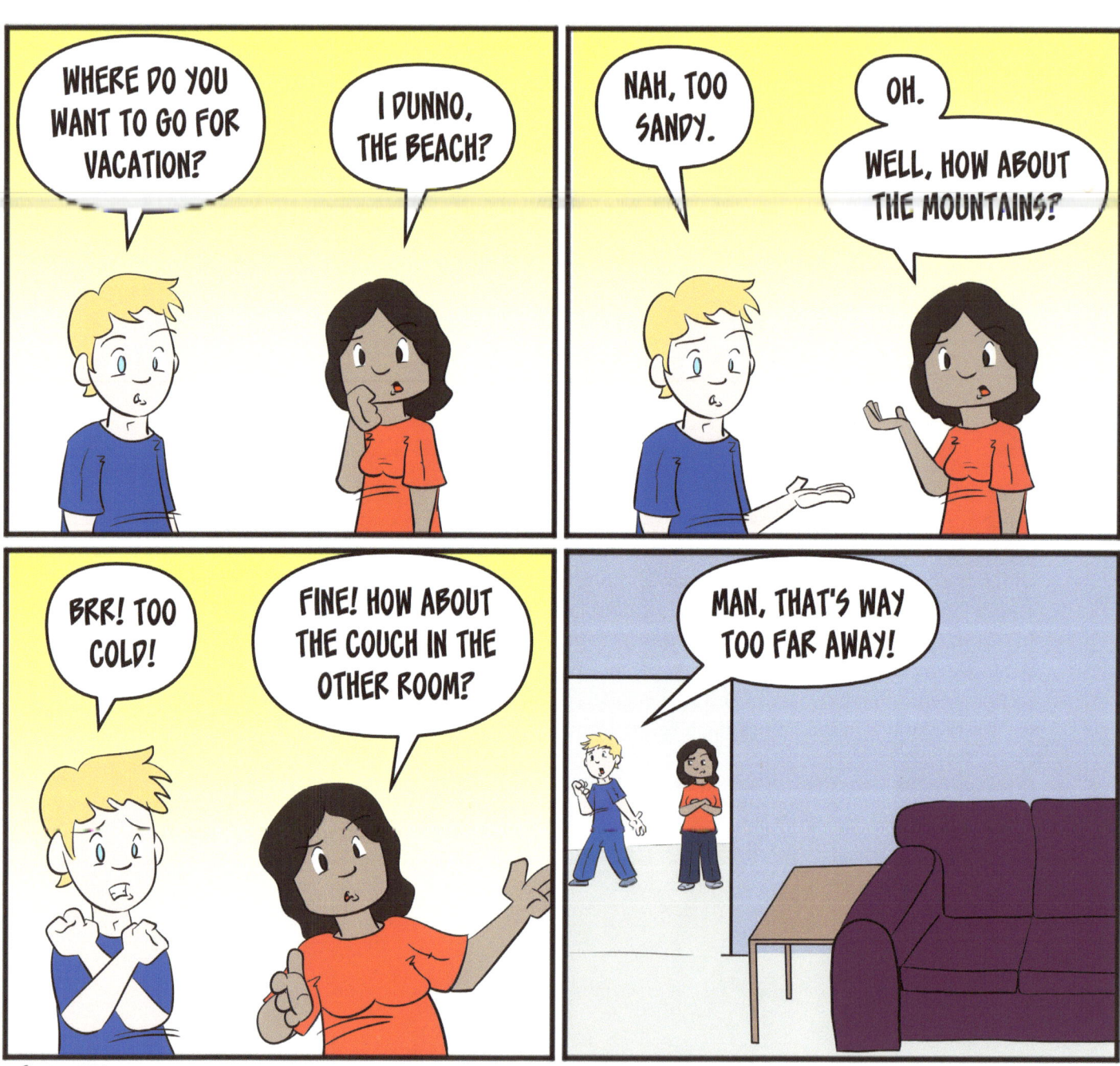

The thing I learned about having this is that my boobs don't define who I am as a person. As a matter of fact, maybe now people will pay attention more to me than my chest!

I thought my male buddies would make fun of me for having breast cancer...instead they all get screened for it regularly. I never thought I would be a breast cancer superhero - but I'm willing to wear the costume...as long as it comes with a cool cape!

I never even considered that I had breasts until I was diagnosed with breast cancer. Now, I'm in remission and happy to welcome them as part of my body as a man!

I didn't have boobs until I was a teenager and those early years were the best of my life. Now I've gone through this...and my best years are still ahead of me!

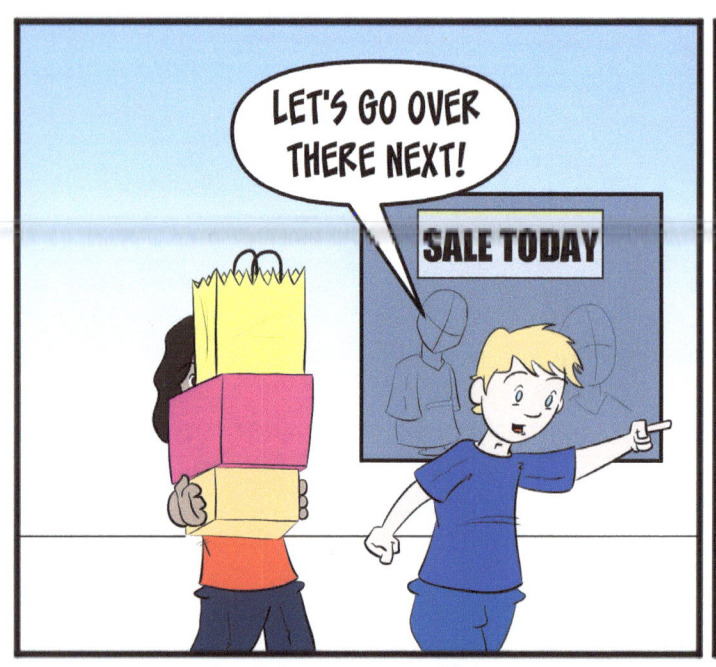
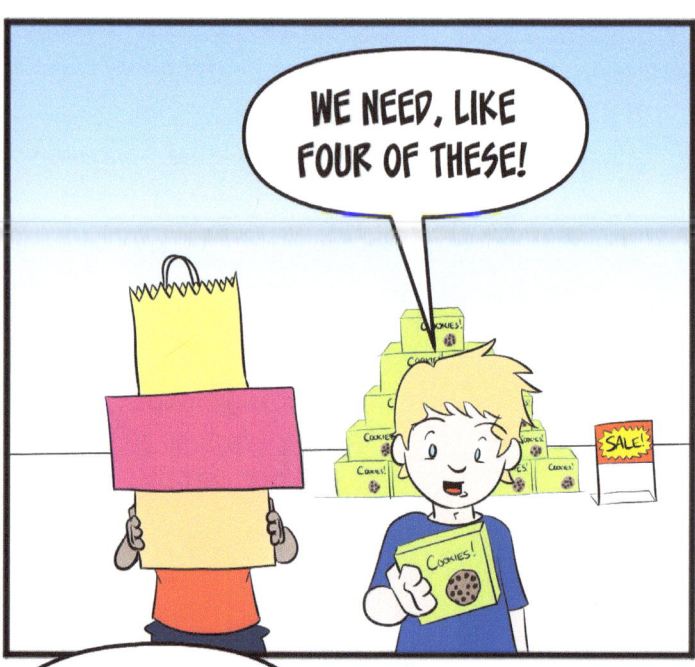
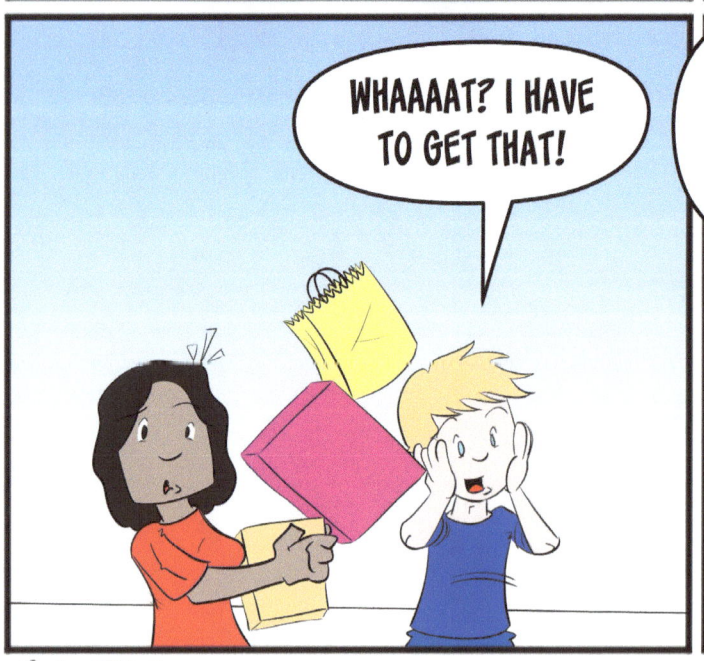
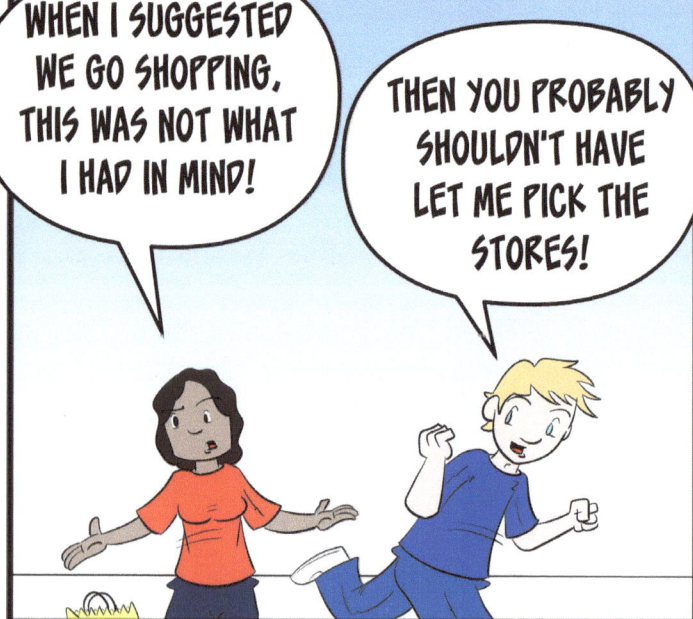

SPIRIT ANIMALS
6

Spirit animals are thought to carry meaning, wisdom, and power. Animals are omnipresent in our lives whether they are pets or live in the wild, yet we often lack a clear understanding of their symbolic nature and what they could mean. When we relate to the spirit of animals, they may offer us powerful insight. In the world of spirit animals, animals can symbolize parts of your personality, skills that you have cultivated successfully or have yet to develop, or a situation or emotions that have recently arisen. Spirit animals can offer guidance, an intuitive understanding that the animals are mostly known for.

For this book purpose, the spirit animal is meant to symbolize a strength that you may wish to reflect upon as your thrive and survive your fight against cancer! Color the spirit animal to symbolize your mood or simply your preference of color.

Free website to find spirit animal quiz - http://www.spiritanimal.info/spirit-animal-quiz/. Also there is a store to buy jewelry at Spirit Animal http://www.spiritanimal.info/.

EAGLE

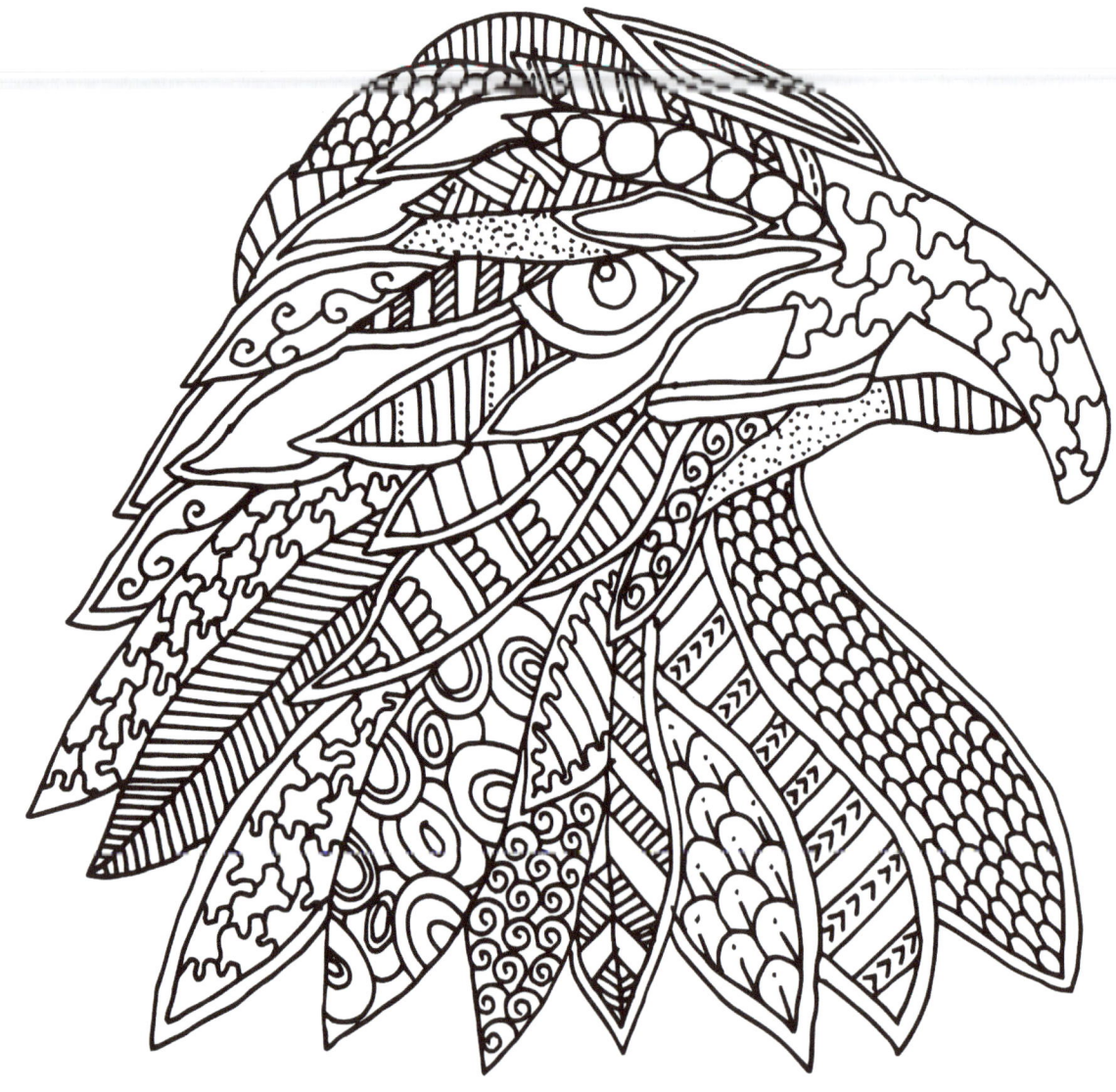

Eagle - HEALING, STRENGTH, COURAGE

Reflection on how I relate to this spirit animal

_____

_____

_____

_____

_____

_____

_____

_____

_____

_____

_____

_____

Tiger - WILLPOWER, STRENGTH, AND HEALTH

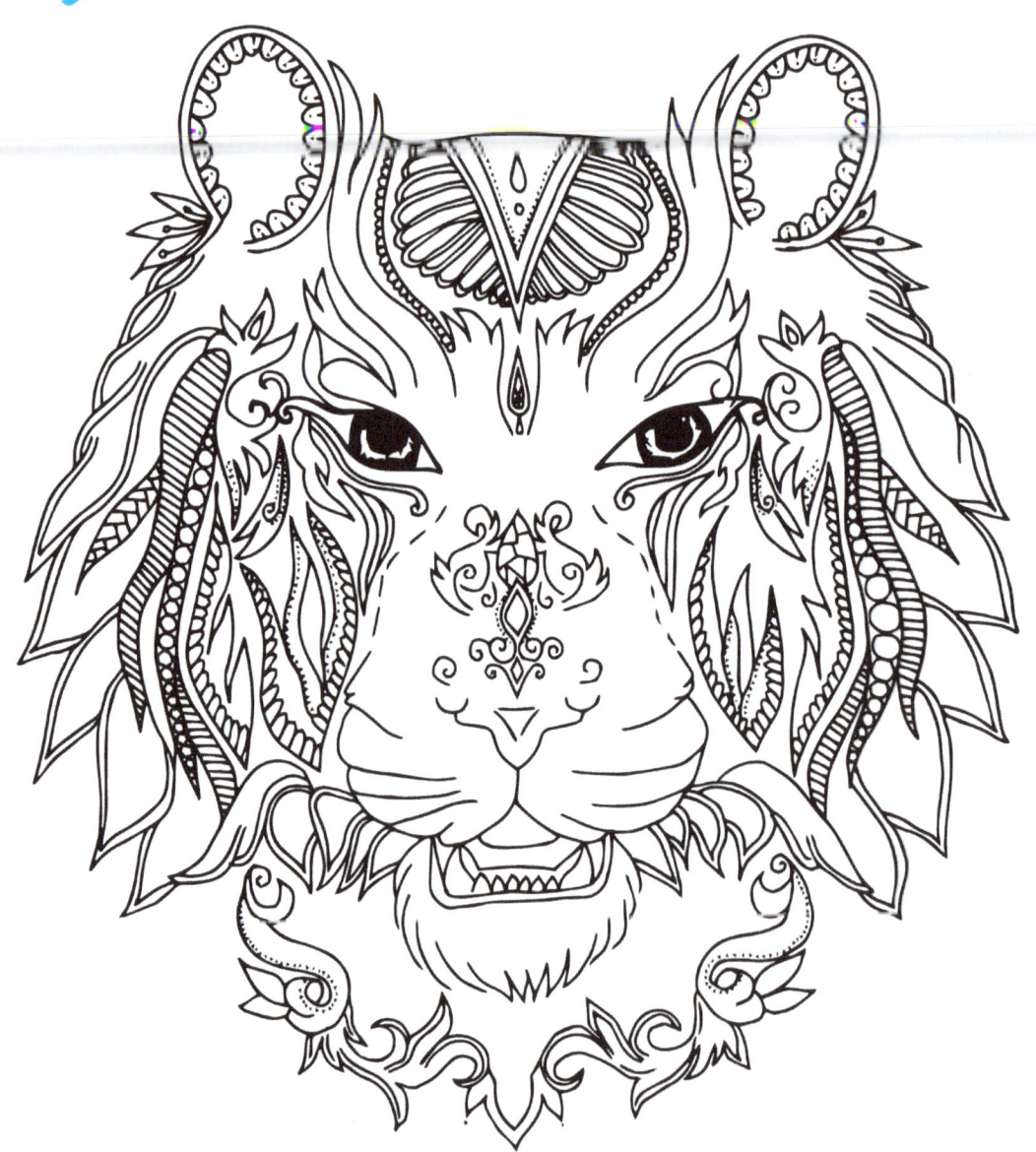

Tiger

Reflection on how I relate to this spirit animal

Turtle - DETERMINATION, WISDOM EMOTIONAL STRENGTH

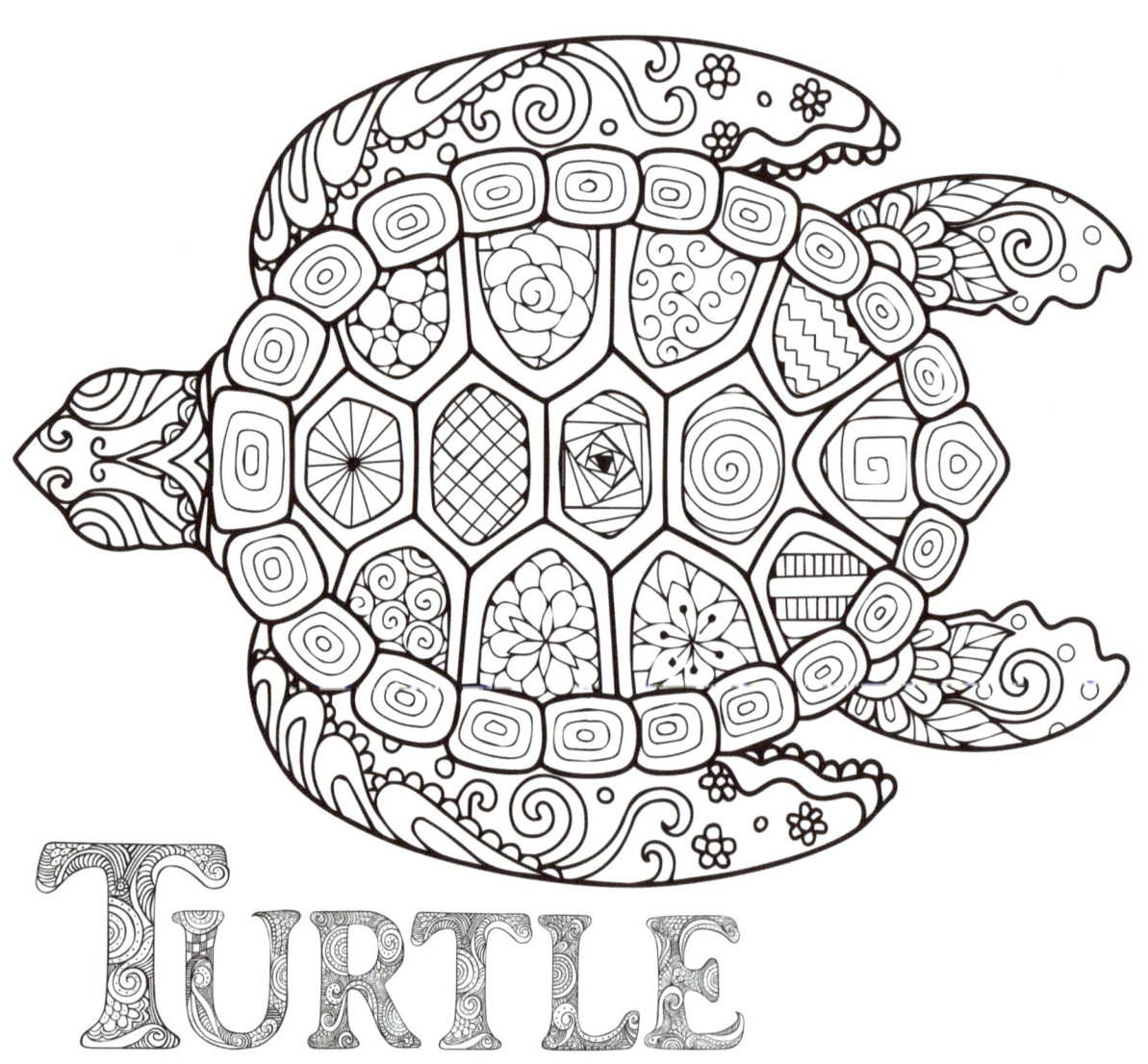

Reflection on how I relate to this spirit animal

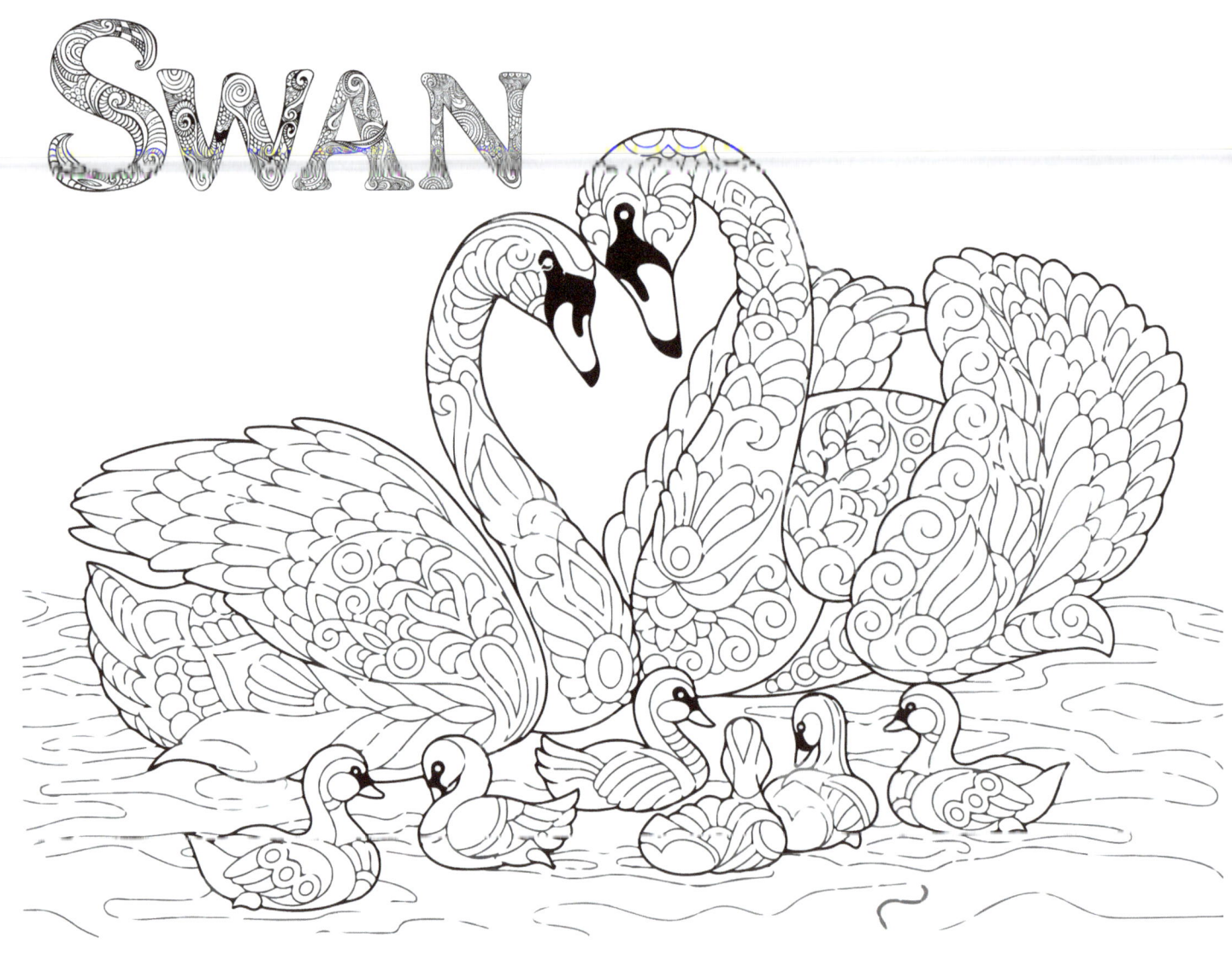

Swan - INNER BEAUTY, GRACE, LOVE

Reflection on how I relate to this spirit animal

Butterfly -RENEWAL, TRANSFORMATION, PLAYFULNESS

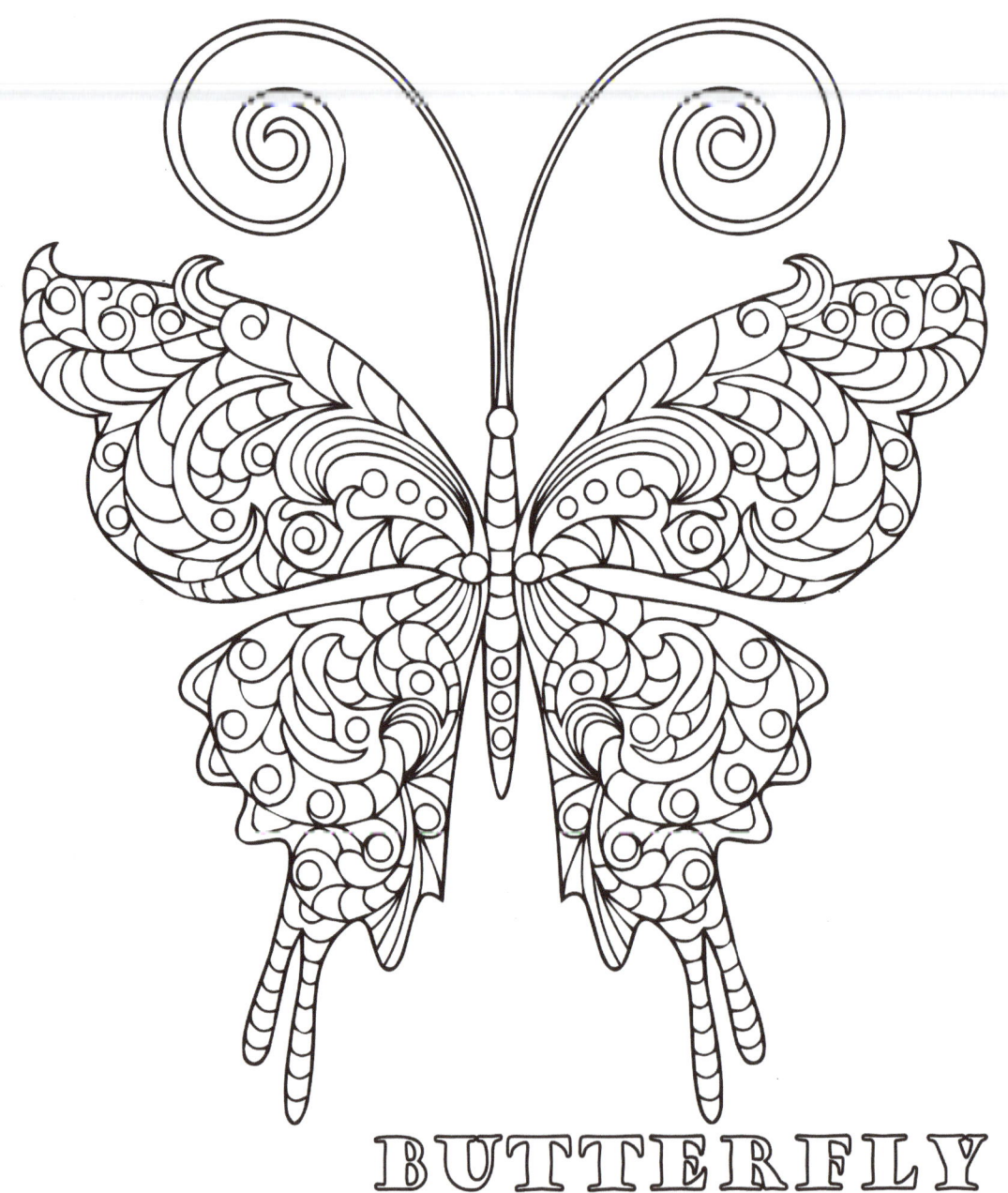

BUTTERFLY

Reflection on how I relate to this spirit animal

Hummingbird - JOY, ADAPTABILITY, RESILIENCY

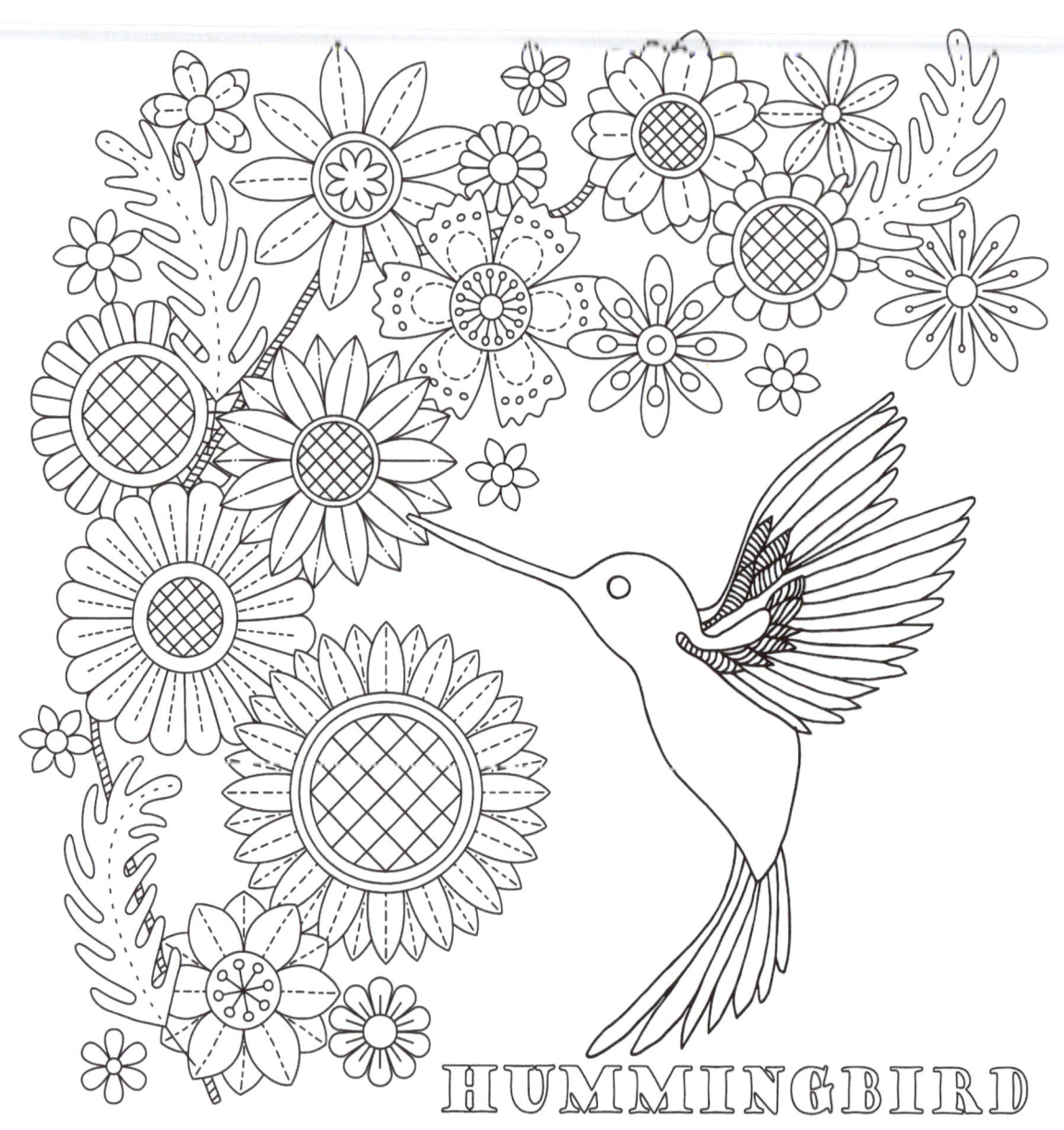

Reflection on how I relate to this spirit animal

BEAR

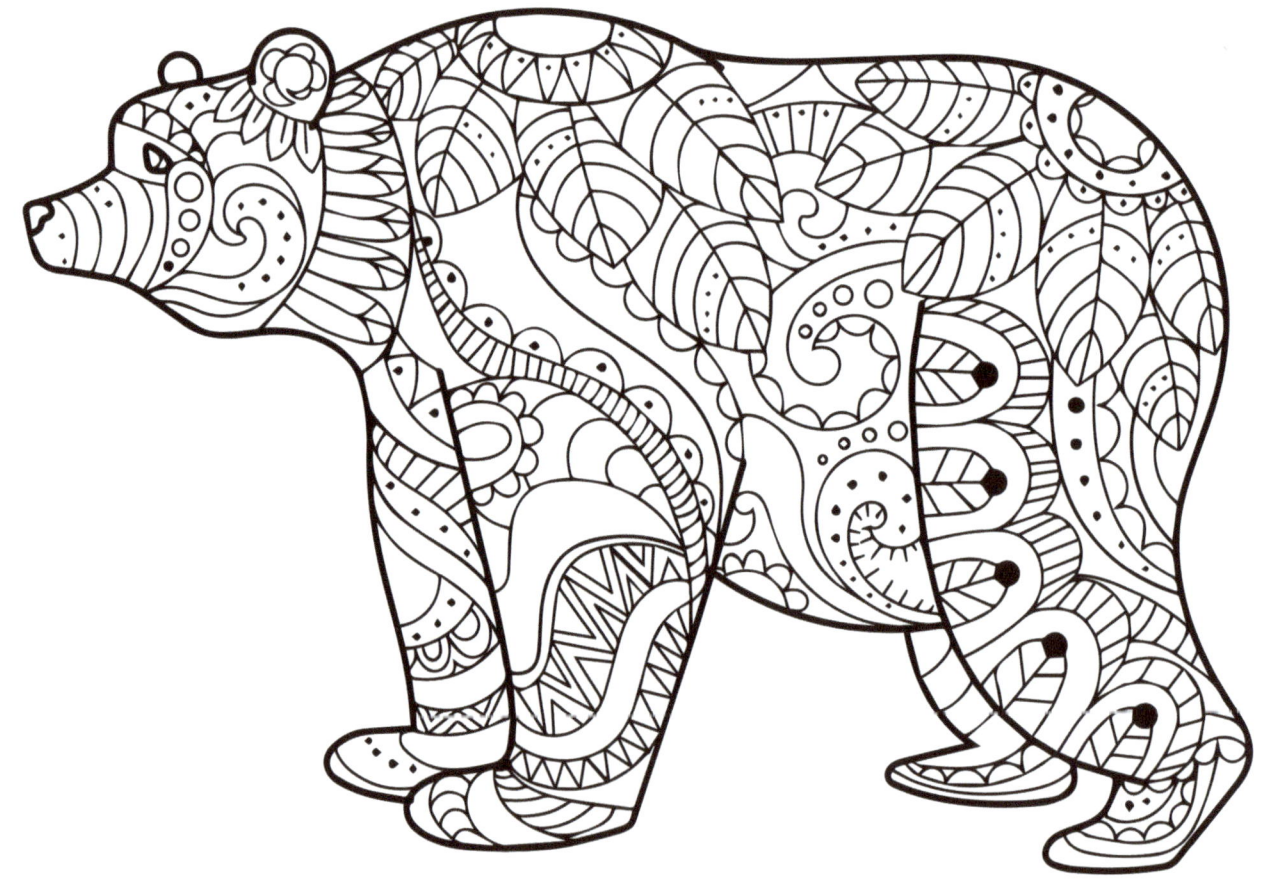

Bear -STRENGTH, CONFIDENCE, HEALING

Reflection on how I relate to this spirit animal

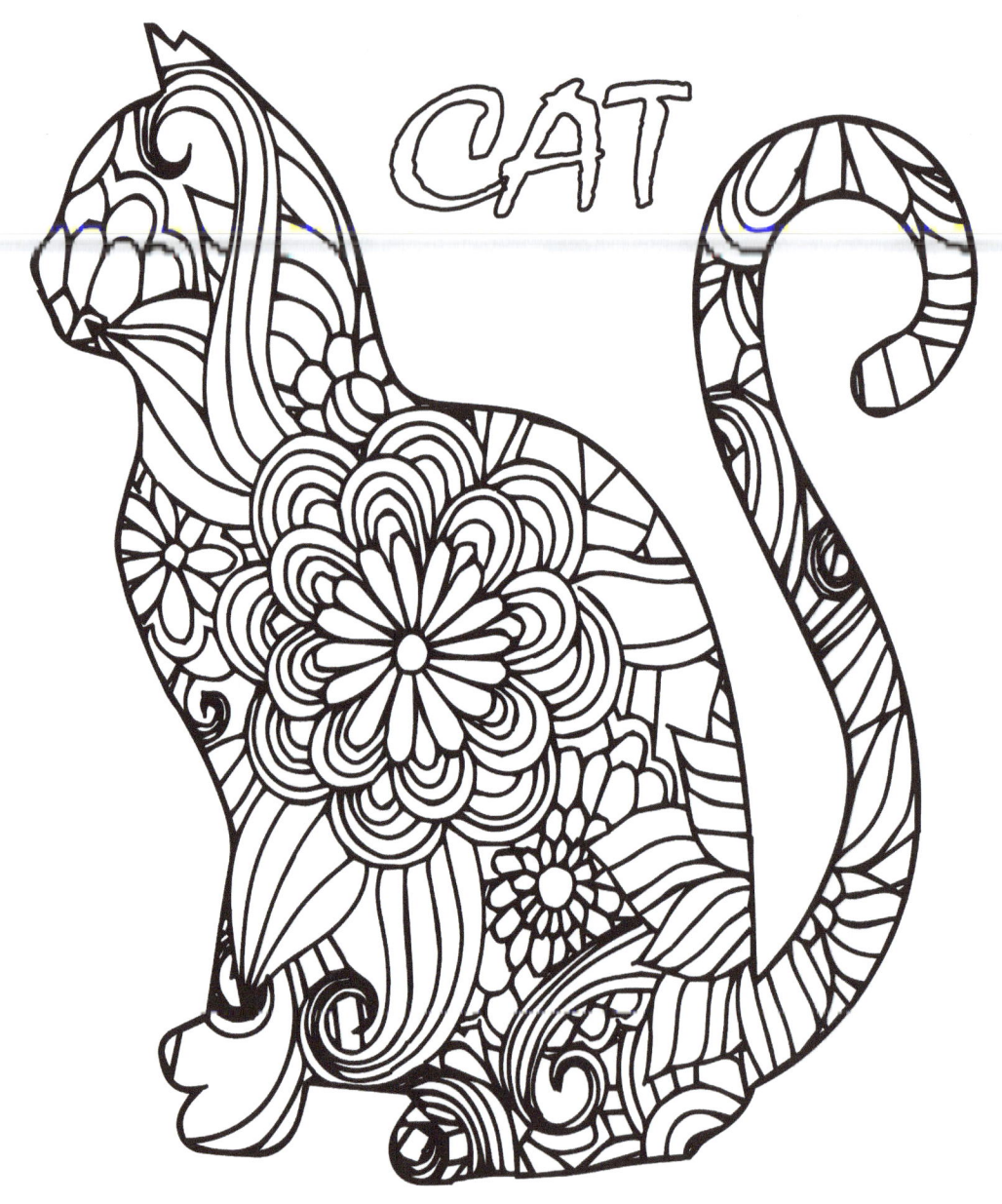

Cat -PATIENCE, COURAGE, HEALING

Reflection on how I relate to this spirit animal

_____

_____

_____

_____

_____

_____

_____

_____

_____

_____

_____

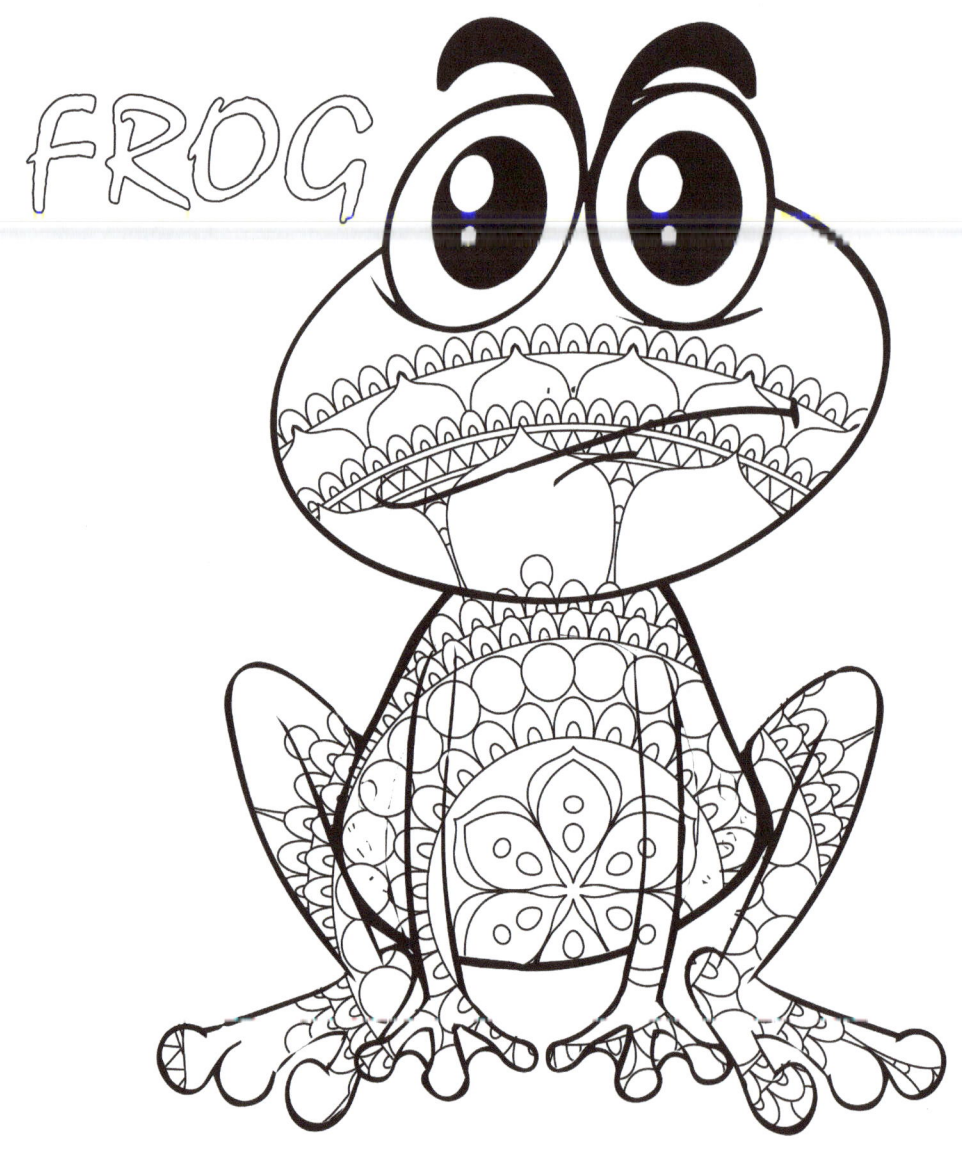

Frog -REBIRTH, CLEANSING, TRANSFORMATION

Reflection on how I relate to this spirit animal

Note: Spirit animal colorable t-shirts are available at the VCS Retail Store at www.zazzle.com/vcs

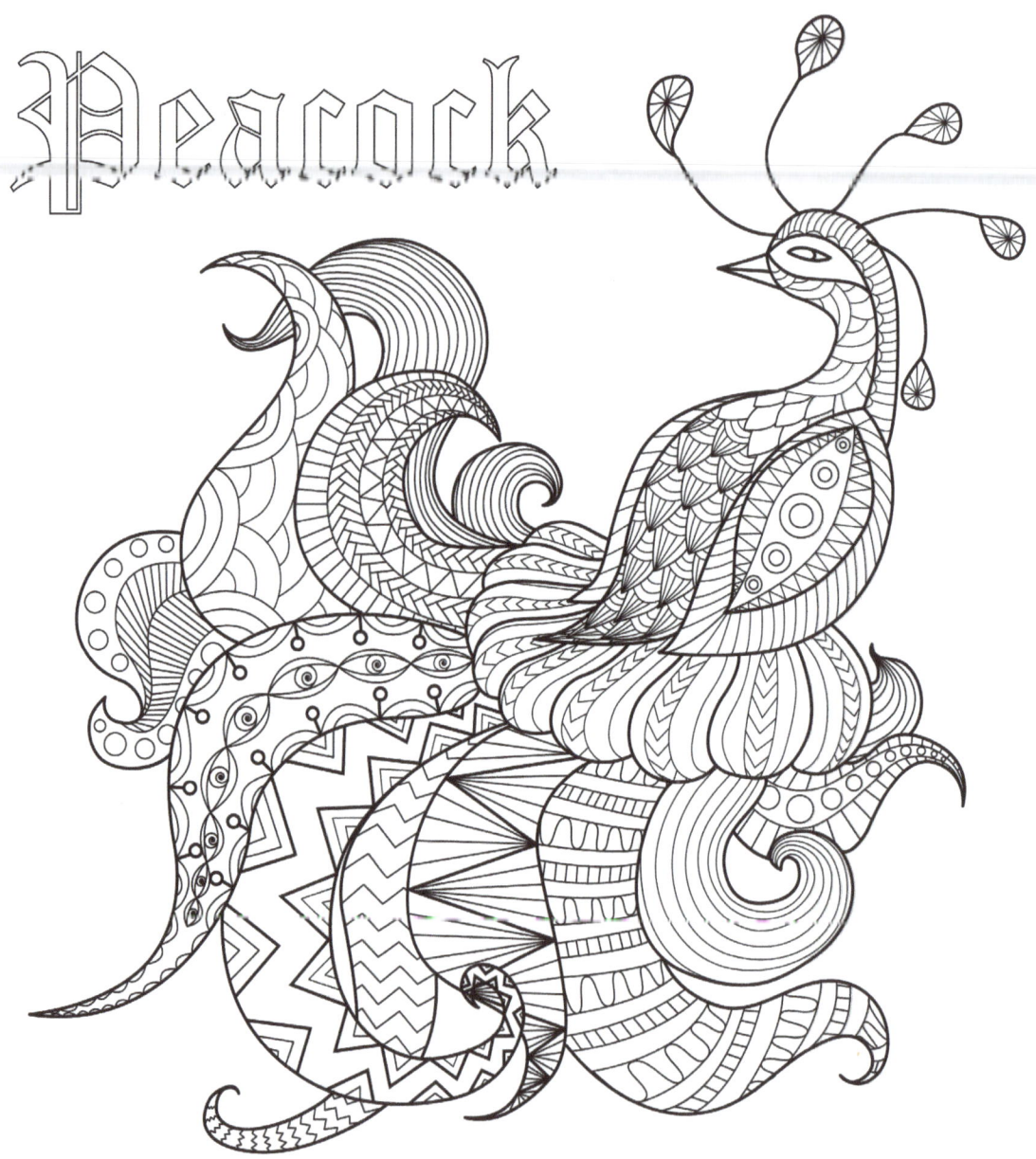

Peacock -BEAUTY, SPIRITUALITY, BALANCE

Reflection on how I relate to this spirit animal

SCRIPTURES
7

Bible verses are great for inspiration, comfort and peace of mind during challenging times. My hope and prayer are that these Bible verses inspire, encourage and build up your most holy faith. The scriptures were taken from various versions of the bible.

Disclaimer: if you do not take part in scripture reading, please feel free to skip this section of the book.

"These things I have spoken to you, so that in Me you may have peace. In the world you have tribulation, but take courage; I have overcome the world."
-John 16:33

"Cast your burden on the Lord [releasing the weight of it] and He will sustain you; He will never allow the [consistently] righteous to be moved (made to slip, fall, or fail)."
-Psalm 55:22 (AMP)

"Do not fear, for I am with you; do not anxiously look about you, for I am your God. I will strengthen you, surely I will help you, surely I will uphold you with My righteous right hand."
-Isaiah 41:10

"I have set the Lord continually before me; because He is at my right hand, I shall not be moved."
-Psalm 16:8 (AMP)

For God did not give us a spirit of timidity (of cowardice, of craven and cringing and fawning fear), but [He has given us a spirit] of power and of love and of calm and well-balanced mind and discipline and self-control.
-2 Tim 1:7 (AMP)

"God is our refuge and strength, a very present help in trouble. Therefore we will not fear, though the earth should change and though the mountains slip into the heart of the sea; though its waters roar and foam, though the mountains quake at its swelling pride. Selah. The LORD of hosts is with us; the God of Jacob is our stronghold. Selah. ."
-Psalm 46:1-3,7

The Lord is good, a Strength and Stronghold in the day of trouble; He knows (recognizes, has knowledge of, and understands) those who take refuge and trust in Him.
-Nahum 1:7 (AMP)

Casting the whole of your care [all your anxieties, all your worries, all your concerns, once and for all] on Him, for He cares for you affectionately and cares about you watchfully.
-1 Peter 5:7 (AMP)

"It is good to give thanks to the Lord, to sing praises to your name, O Most High; to declare your steadfast love in the morning, and your faithfulness by night."
-Psalms 92:1-2 ESV

"Oh give thanks to the Lord, for he is good, for his steadfast love endures forever."
-Psalms 107:1 ESV

"In peace I will both lie down and sleep; for you alone, O Lord, make me dwell in safety."
-Psalms 4:8 ESV

"From the rising of the sun to its setting, the name of the Lord is to be praised."
-Psalms 113:3 ESV

"The steadfast of mind You will keep in perfect peace, Because he trusts in You.
-Isaiah 26:3

Scriptures that inspire you...

Words of faith that build you up...

MINDFUL MEDITATION
8

Meditation is the best way to mentally reduce stress and develop an air of peace and tranquility. Meditation is mindfulness which comes from the Buddhist tradition. It is all about acknowledging reality by letting the mind wander, accepting any thoughts that come up, and understanding the present.

The practice is done by sitting with eyes closed, crossed legs, the back straight, and attention placed on breathing in and out. For the period of meditation, the individual focuses on his or her breathing, and when wandering thoughts emerge, one returns to focusing on the object of meditation, breathing. A consistent practice of mindfulness can reduce anxiety, depression, and perceived distress.

TEN STEPS TO MINDFULNESS MEDITATION

Create time & space.
Choose a regular time each day for mindfulness meditation practice, ideally a quiet place free from distraction

Set a timer.
Start with just 5 minutes and ease your way up to 15-40 minutes.

Find a comfortable sitting position.
Sit cross-legged on the floor, on the grass, or in a chair your feet flat on the ground.

Check your posture.
Sit up straight, hands in a comfortable position. Keep neck long, chin tilted slightly downward, tongue resting on roof of mouth. Relax shoulders. Close eyes or gaze downward 5-10 feet in front of you.

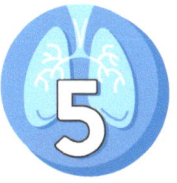
Take deep breaths.
Deep breathing helps settle the body and establish your presence in the space

Direct attention to your breath.
Focus on a part of the body where the breath feels prominent: nostrils; back of throat; or diaphragm. Try not to switch focus.

Maintain attention to your breath.
As you inhale and exhale, focus on the breath. If attention wanders, return to the breath. Let go of thoughts, feelings or distractions.

Repeat steps 6-7.
For the duration of meditation session. The mind will wander. Simply acknowledge this and return to your breath.

Be kind to yourself.
Don't be upset if focus occasionally drifts or if you fall asleep. If very tired, meditate with eyes open and rearrange posture to more erect (but still relaxed) position.

Prepare for a soft landing.
When the timer goes off, keep eyes closed until you're ready to open them. Be thankful. Acknowledge your practice with gratitude.

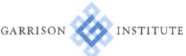

There are two mindfulness exercises for you to practice, if you choose to do so. There is also a 40 minute guided mindful meditations available for purchase from cdbaby.com, amazon app stores, spotify, and other online music stores. You can download it to your device for your listening pleasure. The album consist of the following tracks: Sleep, Relaxation, Positive Energy, and Renewal Meditations. There are 10 easy steps to mindfulness mediation illustrated in the following diagram, with permission give "Courtesy of the Garrison Institute."

STEP BY STEP MINDFULNESS

1. Recognize that there is always time to pause. If only for a moment. And by doing so, you benefit yourself, others and all situations you come into contact with.

2. Relax your gaze or close your eyes.

3. Focus on posture if you're sitting. Body alignment if you're lying down. Shoulders dropped and back. Get as comfortable as you can.

4. Focus on your breathing. Deep inhale in, feeling the belly expand, not the chest. Exhale all the way out. Repeat several times.

5. Release all the muscles in your body, beginning with your face and piece by piece let go of all the tension all the way down to your toes.

6. Begin to engage your senses. What do you feel? Hear? What is the atmosphere around you like? Be present in this moment.

7. Bring your awareness to your inside world. How do you feel? Physically, emotionally?

8. Place a smile on your face and know that all is as it should be. Flow with it.

9. Your practice can be as simple and short or as long and intricate as you desire.

10. Repeat any time you feel overwhelmed, at a loss or upset in any way.

ROOTS

Find a comfortable position, either sitting or lying down. Somewhere you can relax for a moment. Take a deep breath, in through your nose, filling your belly and with the exhale, release all the tension in your body. Close your eyes.

Continue focusing on your breathing. In through the nose, expanding the belly and with each exhale, you're releasing a little more tension, a little more stress and relaxing a little more into your seat. Feeling the heaviness of your body tether you to the earth more and more with each breath. You are grounded.

Bring your attention to your surroundings. What do you hear? What sensations do you feel? Is it hot or cold? What is the atmosphere like? Is it friendly and inviting? Is the energy vibrant or stale? There's no need to attach a judgment or story to any of it. We're not trying to change any of it. Only notice it. We're practicing our awareness. Appreciating all that is, as it is.

There's nothing to do now but take a moment for yourself. You deserve a moment of peace and relaxation so that you may better interact with this brilliant world. We have to care for ourselves before we can care for any one or any thing else properly.

Think of where you are sitting in relation to the whole of the Earth. How magnificent it is to be a part of something so grand. Feel the love and connectedness you have for this existence seep from your heart, a beautiful green mist of energy, spilling from your body until it encompasses not only your entire being but grows to cover the entire planet.

You are an important piece to this machine of life. Playing a part that no one else can play in a plan too grand and complex to understand. Trust in yourself to be led to exactly where you need to be. Embrace that which you are led to with an open mind and an open heart. Interacting with everyone and everything in kindness and compassion for the benefit of all life, including your own.

Bring your awareness back to your body, leaving the green mist to encompass the whole planet in love.

Focusing again on your breathing. See the air around you as a purple mist. As you breathe it in, you notice how fresh, revitalizing and calming it is. You feel yourself becoming even more relaxed and energized as it fills your entire body. Not being exhaled but collecting within to grow through your entire being.

Once it's filled you to the inner depths of your soul, it begins to creep downward, into the earth. Tethering you to it. You see a weblike network beneath the surface of the planet. Like roots running from a tree, everywhere. Follow the roots upward and you notice they're connected to every living man, woman and creature. They're all walking about their lives, unaware of the roots that connect them to one another and the planet. You see it though. All of the billions of connections to one another and each thing. We are all one.

Smile to yourself as you've witnessed such a magnificent thing. Through these roots you draw all of the energy you need from others and from the earth. Lightning strikes the earth every minute, charging us all, providing us with all of the energy we need to live vibrantly. There is an abundance to go around. We need only to tap into its power and invite it in.

Positive energy flows more fluidly than negative. From here on out, we only allow positive energy within our orbit. Any negative energy is repealed and cast away from us. You are finally free from the heavy negative energy that's been dragging you down.

Know that from now on, when you feel stressed, overwhelmed or sick, you can invite this shimmering purple energy up through your roots and allow it to relax you. The more we practice inviting it up, the easier it will become. Every time we ask it to relax us, it will do so more until we are only ever at peace and ease. Light and happy, only ever full of positive energy and vibrations. Until we eventually need it no more but can produce relaxation and happiness not only for ourselves, but for others as well.

Stay here as long as you need soaking up the endless amount of loving energy. When you're ready, smile to yourself, having experienced such a brilliant secret to this magical world we live in. Continue about your day holding onto this energy, protecting it as your own and only giving what you can spare. Just by existing in this state, you're a positive influence on the world and others. No else is needed. You are enough.

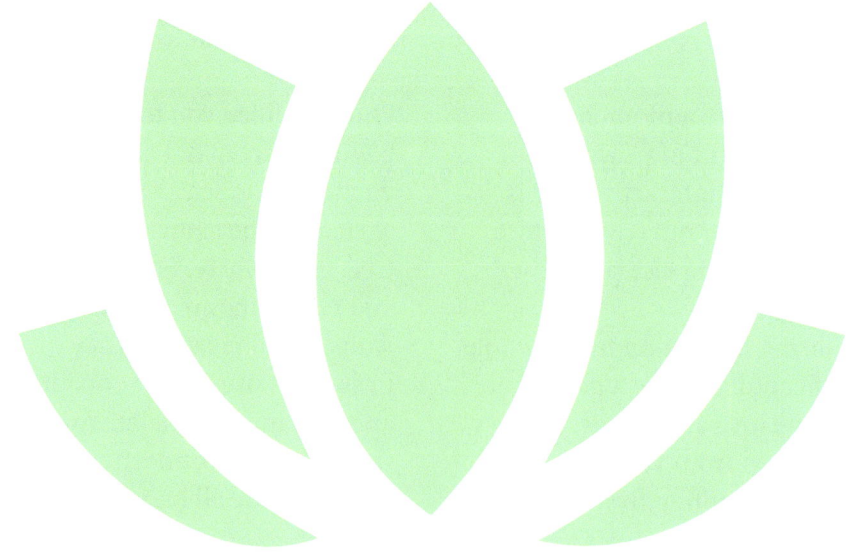

LIGHT

Find a comfortable position either sitting or lying down. If you're sitting, correct your posture. Shoulders back and down, Spine straight and stretched tall. If you're lying down, make sure you're straight and in alignment. Close your eyes. Feel your body sink into your seat, allowing yourself to give it all of your weight, trusting it to hold you. There's nothing to do right now. You deserve a few moments to yourself, for yourself, mind, body and spirit.

As you begin to focus on breathing, you notice that you're surrounded by shimmering white light. As you take a deep breath, inhaling the light through your nose, filling the belly, not the chest, you feel a sense of happiness and peace. It's crisp and refreshing like morning air. It feels alive with the greatest of ambitions.

Hold onto it, counting smoothly to four and then releasing it evenly through the mouth. What's exhaled is not the light. The light remains inside of you and has taken the space in your body of something dark. The darkness has been expelled though your breath. You feel a sense of peace and happiness filling your belly where the light resides. More relaxed with the exhale of the darkness. Like a great relief.
Take another deep breath and this time, see the light go to your feet where it replaces the darkness there, expelling it with your exhale and leaving your feet glowing with a glittery white light that feels magnificently peaceful and relaxed. Warm like a blanket of love.

The next breath fills your legs, leaving them the same way. Every muscle and tendon in them relaxed and at ease. You continue to focus on your breathing, sending the glittering light to every piece of your body, every cell, until you're completely relaxed. Vibrant like sunshine on a crystal. It finds every tiny inkling of darkness that resides in your body and banishes it from you. It cares for you so deeply, pure kindness and compassion. Like all the good that's in the universe here to serve you. Allow the light to work.

Each breath makes you brighter. You feel an overwhelming sense of joy at ridding your body of the darkness. Chasing it away so easily, you can't help but smile for all you have to do is breathe and allow. You feel so much better with the light instead. You hadn't realized how much the darkness was weighing you down. Now, you feel as though you're floating. High on happiness and life. Such a wonderfully intoxicating feeling.

When your body is so full of light that it simply can't hold any more, it continues to be drawn to you with each breath. Like a magnet, it's attaching itself to you. Connecting you to the earth below and the sky above. Creating a shimmering bubble of protection around you and growing until it encompasses all of your family and friends and draws more power and more loving energy from our mother earth. You feel a wholeness. A connectedness to every living being on the planet. You are all one. We are all one.

The darkness is always trying to creep back in. Hold onto your shimmering bubble of light for protection throughout your day. Anytime you feel heavy, stressed or negativity in any way, know that all you have to do is take a few deep breaths of light to feel better.

Make this process your own. Tweak it to your needs, your desires. Spending more time on the places in your body that carry more darkness, in whatever form it may be. Taking as much or as little time as you require to relax yourself with the light. As frequently as you need.

The more you practice, the easier it will be, the more natural it will become until you're doing it automatically. No darkness is welcome here.

We don't mention sickness or cancer because naming it gives it power. That which we focus on grows. We only want to focus on healing.

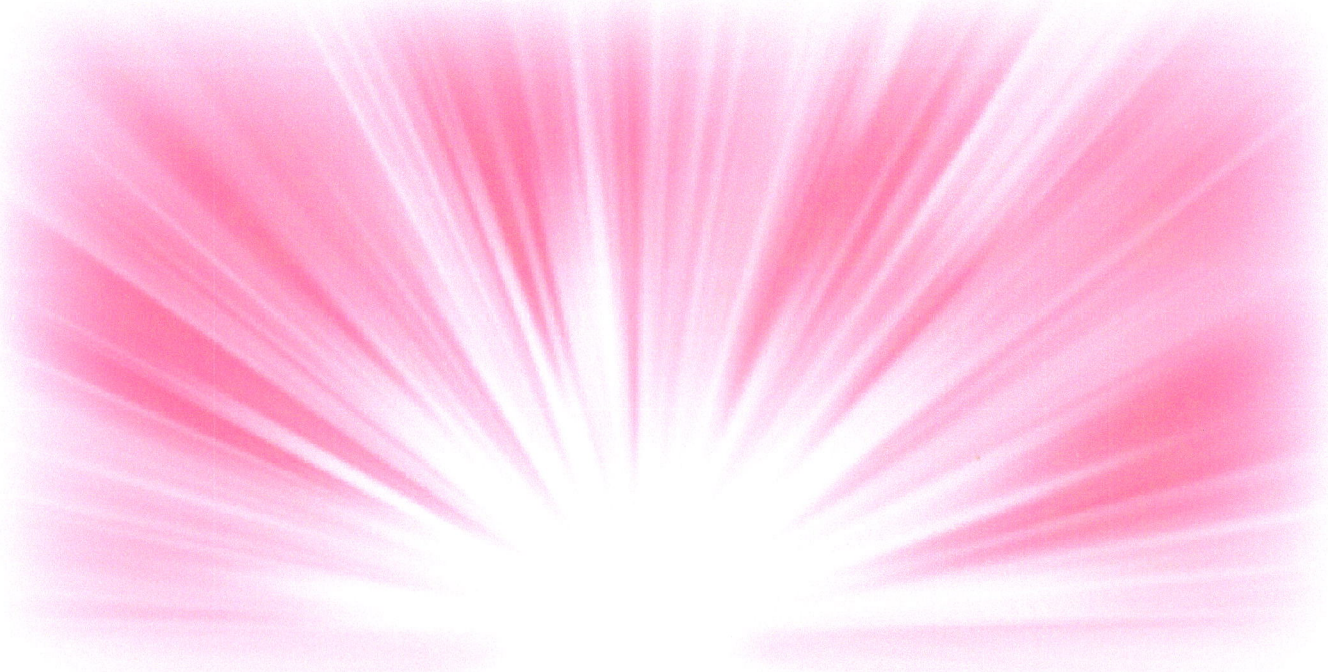

ORGANIZATION WEBSITES

10

There are a plethora of national and local organizations to assist you with your fight against cancer. I have listed a few websites that have comprehensive resources for many forms of cancer and topics. *Please use your own discretion when viewing websites and their information for creditability and reliability of the information and sources.*

Visit the B.O.P Cancer social media page for information posts about cancer care, the B.O.P Cancer book series, retail store, and cancer awareness events.

- American Cancer Society- www.cancer.org
- Susan G. Komen- https://ww5.komen.org/
- Cancer Care- www.cancercare.org
- BreastCancer.org- www.breastcancer.org
- American Breast Cancer Foundation- www.abcf.org
- Natinal Breast Cancer Foundation- www.nationalbreastcancer.org
- National Foundation for Cancer Research- www.nfcr.org
- Cancer Research Foundation- www.cancerresroucefoundation.org
- Headcovers Unlimited- https://www.headcovers.com/blog/american-cancer-society-wigs/
- Brenda's Brown Bossom Buddies- http://brendasbrownbosombuddies.org/
- Joy of Life Foundation- https://joytolifefoundation.org/
- Triple Negative Breast Cancer Foundation- https://tnbcfoundation.org/
- Young Survivor Coalition- https://www.youngsurvival.org/

Please donate to the Dr. Tomeka D. Russell, MD foundation. The foundation grants scholarships to students for going to college to study science that targets cancer.

Appendix

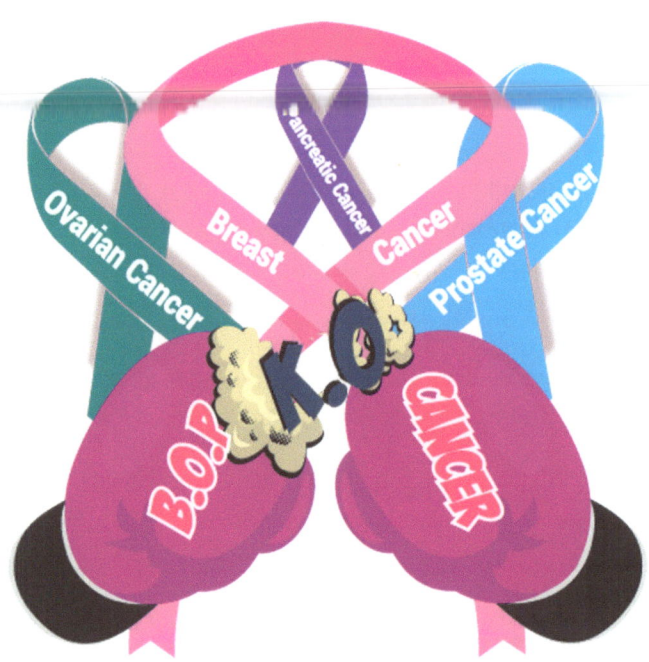

Practice Preventive Healthcare: Check your Breast Monthly
Let's BOP Cancer (***knock out***) through early detection!

Monthly Self Breast Exam ➤

MALE

IN THE SHOWER: Step 1. Place your right hand behind your head to examine your right breast. **2.** Check for lumps, knots, or thickenings by using either the Up and Down, Circle, or Wedge pattern with the left hand three middle finger pads. **3.** While checking the breast apply variation in pressure using in this order, light, medium, then firm pressure in overlapping, dime-size circular motions to fill the breast tissue and underarm. **4.** Check for lumps and thickenings in the breasts **5.** Repeat the steps on the left breast by placing your left hand behind your head, checking with your right hand following steps 2-4.

BEFORE A MIRROR: Step 1: Place your hands on your hips **2.** Press your hands firmly down on your hips, **3.** Check the breast for the following changes: size, shape, and skin texture of the breasts; and **4.** Check the nipples of your breasts for usual discharge.

SITTING or STANDING: Step 1. Slightly raise one of your arm and exam each underarm for lump. **2.** Repeat this step with the opposite arm.

LYING DOWN: Position your self in bed to allow an even distribution of the breast tissue. **Step 1.** Place your right hand behind your head to examine your right breast. **2.** Check for lumps, knots, or thickenings by using either the Up and Down, Circle, or Wedge pattern with the left hand three middle finger pads. **3.** While checking the breast apply variation in pressure using in this order, light, medium, then firm pressure in overlapping, dime-size circular motions to fill the breast tissue and underarm. **4.** Check for lumps and thickenings in the breasts **5.** Repeat the steps on the left breast by placing your left hand behind your head, checking with your right hand following steps 2-4.

FEMALE

IN THE SHOWER: Step 1. Place your right hand behind your head to examine your right breast. **2.** Check for lumps, knots, or thickenings by using either the Up and Down, Circle, or Wedge pattern with the left hand three middle finger pads. **3.** While checking the breast apply variation in pressure using in this order, light, medium, then firm pressure in overlapping, dime-size circular motions to fill the breast tissue and underarm. **4.** Check for lumps and thickenings in the breasts **5.** Repeat the steps on the left breast by placing your left hand behind your head, checking with your right hand following steps 2-4.

BEFORE THE MIRROR: Step 1: Place your hands on your hips **2.** press your hands firmly down on your hips, **3.** Check the breast for the following changes: size, shape, and skin texture of the breasts; and **4.** Check the nipples of your breasts for usual discharge.

SITTING OR STANDING: Step 1. Slightly raise one of your arm and exam each underarm for lump. **2.** Repeat this step with the opposite arm.

LYING DOWN: Step 1. Place your right hand behind your head to examine your right breast. **2.** Check for lumps, knots, or thickenings by using either the Up and Down, Circle, or Wedge pattern with the left hand three middle finger pads. **3.** While checking the breast apply variation in pressure using in this order, light, medium, then firm pressure in overlapping, dime-size circular motions to fill the breast tissue and underarm. **4.** Check for lumps and thickenings in the breasts **5.** Repeat the steps on the left breast by placing your left hand behind your head, checking with your right hand following steps 2-4.

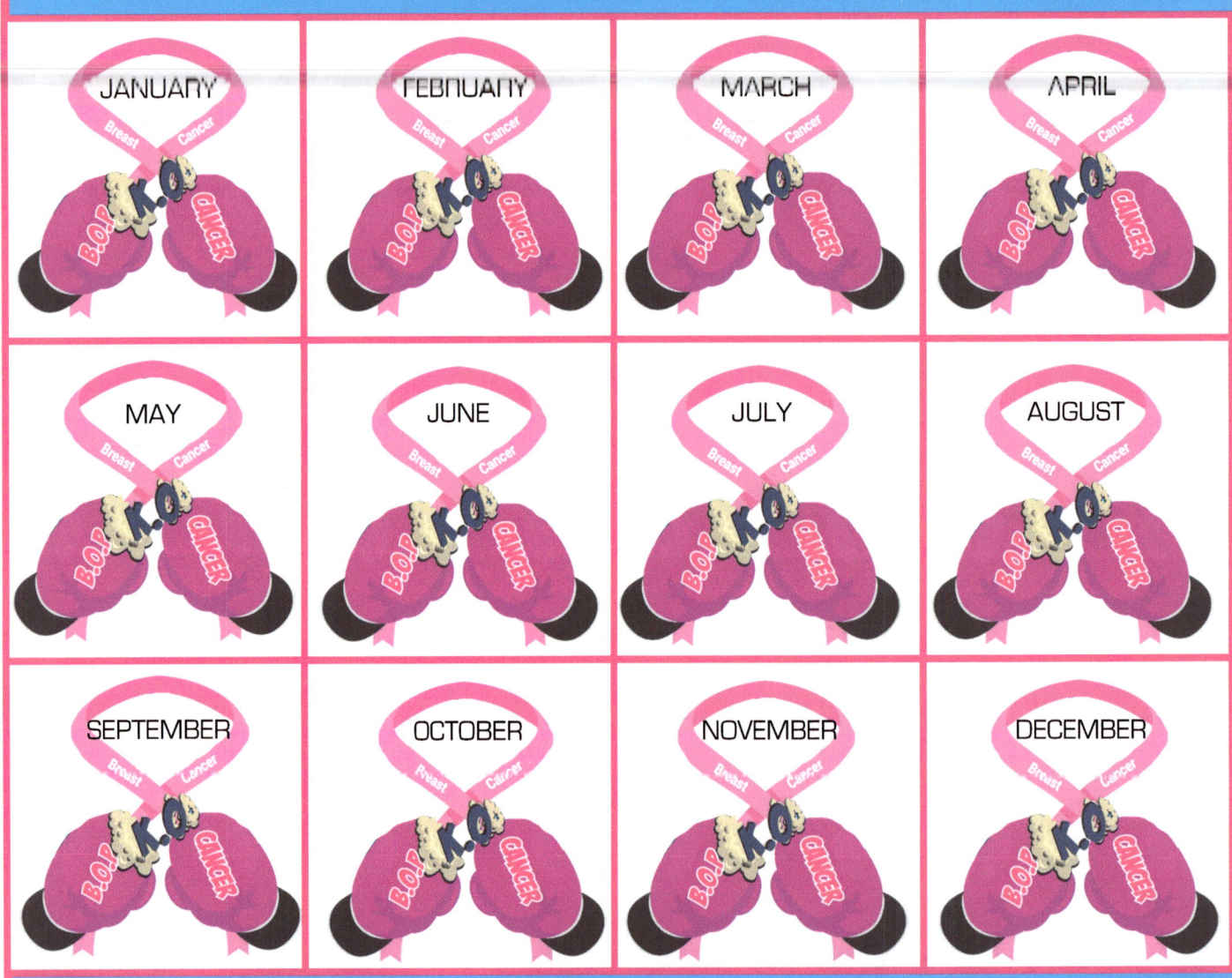

Breast Self-Exam for Him!
Check yourself the same day every month.

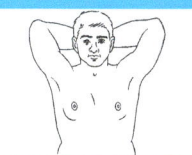 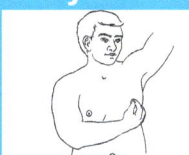 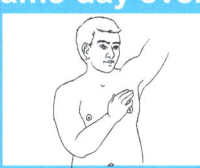 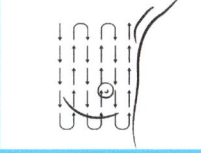

1. Check your breasts in front of a mirror for any symptoms or abnormalities.
2. Examine the nipple, most men find their lumps under the nipple.
3. In a sitting or standing position, use the pads of the three middle fingers - examine using light, medium, and deep pressure. (See step 4, for area to be examined)
4. Examining starts at the collarbone and continues down and up the entire breast in a vertical pattern.

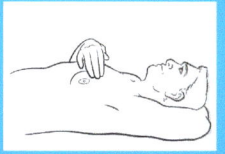

5. Position yourself in bed which leads to a more even distribution of your breast tissue. Repeat step 3 and 4.

Signs and Symptoms

- A painless lump or thickening in your breast tissue.
- Changes to the skin covering your breast, such as dimpling, wrinkling, redness, or scaling.
- Changes to your nipple, such as redness or scaling, or a nipple that begins to turn inward.
- Discharge from your nipple.

 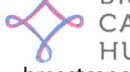

BREAST CANCER HUB — breastcancerhub.org
SARAH CANNON Cancer Institute — hcamidwest.com
The Male Breast Cancer Coalition — malebreastcancercoalition.org
Kurlbaum Illustration — kurlbaumillustration.com

Breast Self-Exam for Her!
Check your breasts the same day every month.
Check yourself a week after your period starts when swelling and sensitivity are less.

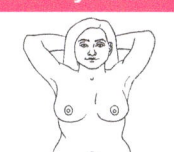 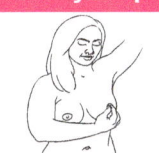 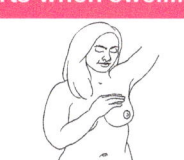 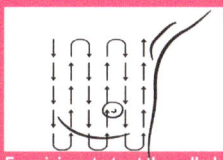

1. Check your breasts in front of a mirror for any symptoms or abnormalities.
2. Check your nipples carefully, lumps may be found behind the nipple.
3. In a sitting or standing position, use the pads of the three middle fingers - examine using light, medium, and deep pressure. (See step 4, for area to be examined)
4. Examining starts at the collarbone and continues down and up the entire breast in a vertical pattern.

5. Position yourself in bed which leads to a more even distribution of your breast tissue. Repeat step 3 and 4.

Signs and Symptoms

- Swelling of all or part of a breast (even if no distinct lump is felt).
- Skin irritation or dimpling (sometimes looking like an orange peel).
- Breast or nipple pain.
- Nipple retraction (turning inward).
- Redness, scaliness, or thickening of the nipple or breast skin.
- Nipple discharge (other than breast milk).

  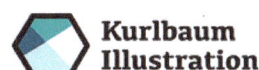

BREAST CANCER HUB
SARAH CANNON Cancer Institute
The Male Breast Cancer Coalition
Kurlbaum Illustration

Signs of Breast Changes

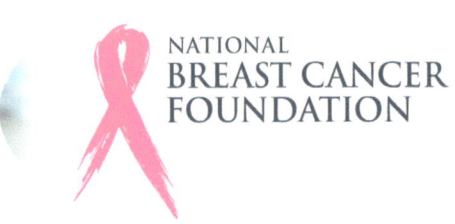

HOW TO CHECK FOR BREAST CANCER

In most cases, changes to the breast aren't due to cancer, but if you notice a change, see your GP as soon as possible.

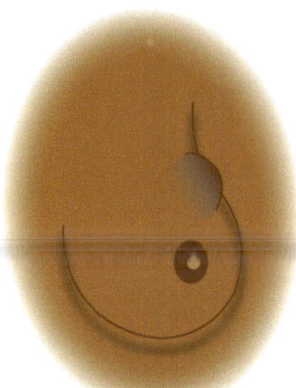

LUMP

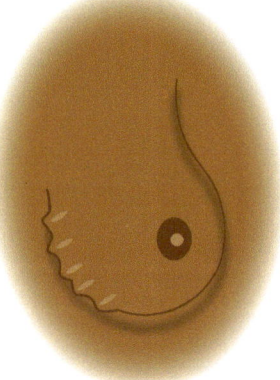

SKIN DIMPLING

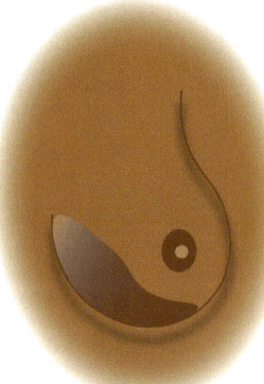

CHANGE IN SKIN COLOR OR TEXTURE

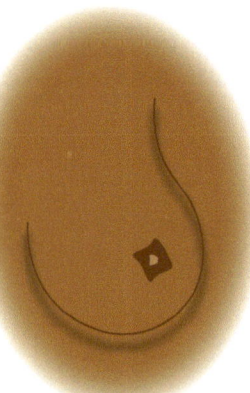

CHANGE IN HOW THE NIPPLE LOOKS (e.g. pulling of the nipple)

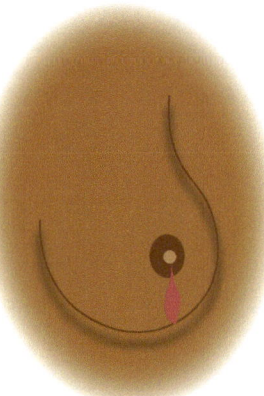

CLEAR OR BLOODY FLUID THAT LEAKS OUT OF THE NIPPLE

Crossword & Sudoku Puzzle Answers

Healthy Eating: Fruits & Vegetables

Good nutrition is to key to any persons healthy eating plan. Have fun and discover foods that are nutritional and tasty!

Across:
- 2. TOMATOES
- 4. PEACHES
- 8. WATERMELON
- 9. CARROTS
- 11. NUTS
- 12. GRAPES
- 14. PEAS
- 15. KALE

Down:
- 1. CABBAGE
- 3. ASPARAGUS
- 5. BROCCOLI
- 6. BERRIES
- 7. ORANGE
- 10. ONION
- 13. APPLE

1

8	7	9	6	2	4	5	1	3
4	1	2	5	7	3	6	9	8
5	3	6	9	1	8	2	7	4
6	4	3	1	9	2	7	8	5
7	2	5	4	8	6	9	3	1
1	9	8	7	3	5	4	2	6
3	8	4	2	6	9	1	5	7
2	5	1	8	4	7	3	6	9
9	6	7	3	5	1	8	4	2

2

3	9	4	6	5	1	7	8	2
2	7	6	3	8	4	1	5	9
5	1	8	9	7	2	3	6	4
8	6	2	5	1	7	9	4	3
1	5	9	4	2	3	6	7	8
4	3	7	8	9	6	2	1	5
7	8	5	1	3	9	4	2	6
6	2	3	7	4	5	8	9	1
9	4	1	2	6	8	5	3	7

3

4	6	5	1	7	3	8	9	2
1	9	2	4	5	8	6	3	7
3	8	7	9	2	6	5	4	1
5	3	6	8	9	7	2	1	4
8	1	9	2	3	4	7	6	5
2	7	4	6	1	5	3	8	9
6	2	3	7	4	1	9	5	8
9	5	1	3	8	2	4	7	6
7	4	8	5	6	9	1	2	3

4

5	3	9	1	6	7	4	8	2
2	8	6	4	3	9	7	1	5
4	1	7	8	2	5	3	6	9
1	7	2	3	8	6	5	9	4
8	6	4	5	9	2	1	7	3
9	5	3	7	1	4	6	2	8
6	4	8	2	7	3	9	5	1
3	9	1	6	5	8	2	4	7
7	2	5	9	4	1	8	3	6

5

4	3	5	1	6	9	8	2	7
2	8	6	7	5	3	9	4	1
9	1	7	2	8	4	5	3	6
7	4	8	9	2	6	3	1	5
3	5	9	8	1	7	4	6	2
6	2	1	3	4	5	7	8	9
5	7	2	6	3	8	1	9	4
1	9	3	4	7	2	6	5	8
8	6	4	5	9	1	2	7	3

6

9	5	3	2	6	8	7	1	4
7	4	2	3	9	1	6	5	8
8	1	6	4	7	5	9	2	3
1	6	9	8	3	4	5	7	2
4	3	7	5	2	9	1	8	6
5	2	8	7	1	6	4	3	9
6	7	4	1	8	2	3	9	5
2	9	1	6	5	3	8	4	7
3	8	5	9	4	7	2	6	1

7

5	4	9	6	7	8	3	2	1
7	8	1	2	4	3	9	5	6
6	2	3	9	5	1	8	7	4
9	7	5	3	6	2	4	1	8
4	3	2	1	8	7	6	9	5
8	1	6	5	9	4	7	3	2
2	6	4	7	1	9	5	8	3
3	5	7	8	2	6	1	4	9
1	9	8	4	3	5	2	6	7

8

8	3	5	6	9	4	1	2	7
2	9	7	3	1	8	4	6	5
4	6	1	5	7	2	9	8	3
1	5	8	2	3	9	7	4	6
9	7	4	1	8	6	3	5	2
6	2	3	7	4	5	8	1	9
7	8	6	9	5	1	2	3	4
3	4	2	8	6	7	5	9	1
5	1	9	4	2	3	6	7	8

1	5	8	6	9	2	4	3	7
7	9	2	5	4	3	6	8	1
3	4	6	1	8	7	5	9	2
4	6	3	2	5	9	1	7	8
9	7	5	8	6	1	2	4	3
2	8	1	3	7	4	9	6	5
8	2	4	9	3	5	7	1	6
5	3	9	7	1	6	8	2	4
6	1	7	4	2	8	3	5	9

9

6	9	2	8	4	1	3	5	7
1	8	4	5	3	7	6	9	2
7	5	3	6	9	2	1	4	8
8	6	1	7	5	3	9	2	4
9	2	5	4	8	6	7	3	1
3	4	7	1	2	9	8	6	5
4	7	6	3	1	5	2	8	9
5	1	9	2	6	8	4	7	3
2	3	8	9	7	4	5	1	6

10

ABOUT THE AUTHOR

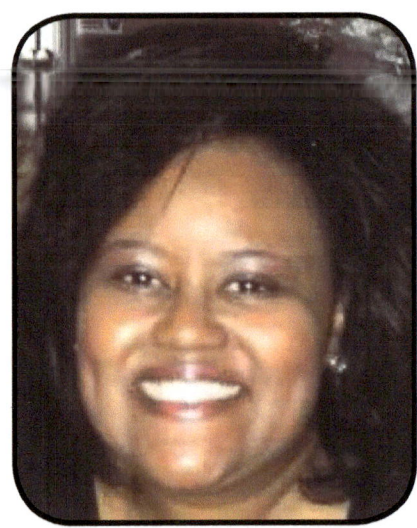

April L. Jones, PhD, LMSW, is a multi-talented social science and business professional, independent researcher, and author from Alabama, USA. She has traveled the world sharing her published studies and books. She was inspired to write the BOP Cancer book series when she lost her beloved cousin to triple negative breast cancer. She also lost her grandfather to prostate cancer and a cousin to pancreatic cancer. Having a friend who is a survivor of ovarian cancer and many others who survivored other forms of cancer, she wanted to target something they all felt was missing with cancer treatment i.e. mental wellness. Being a lifelong social worker and seeing the fight, being a caregiver, and witnessing survivors wonder after ever examination "will it come back?" or "is this illness cancer?" spurred the writing of this book in hope to fill the gap in psychological self-care for those with cancer, caregiving, and survivoring everyday. Dr. Jones hopes this book will inspire you to undertake a journey of mental wellness and continued self-care as a part of your walk with cancer.

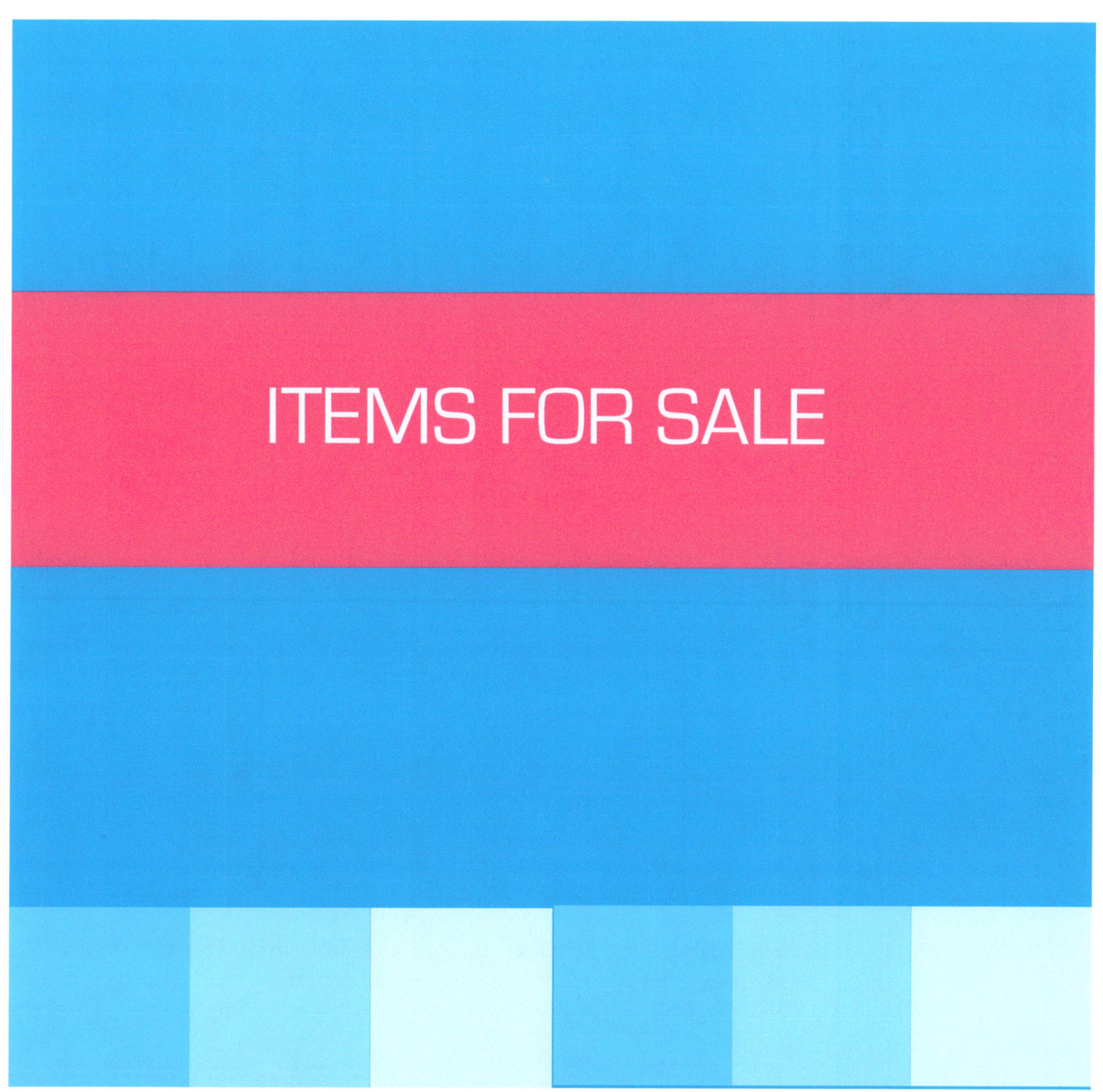

VCS Retail Store

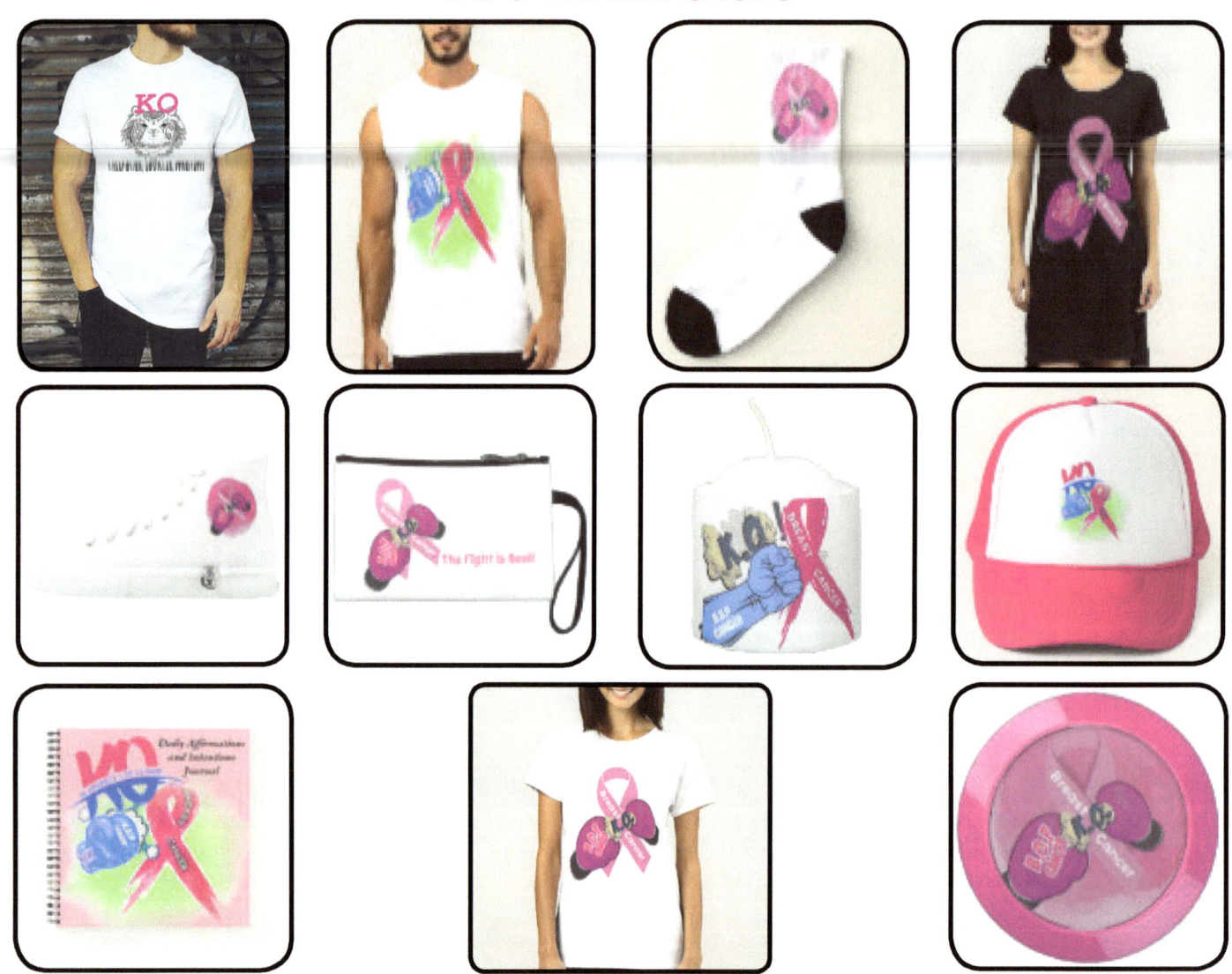

There are daily discounts on the Zazzle store. Fundraiser options are available for the Teespring store at https://teespring.com/stores/vcs-retail-store?aid=marketplace. Interested nonprofits should contact me via email request at vcsllc.co@gmail.com or at the website contact card on www.vcsllc.co.

www.zazzle.com/vcsllc

Book Series & Album Information

The B.O.P Cancer book series consist of three more books available online at all major books stores. You may also get the 40 Minute Guided Mindful Meditations at major music stores online.

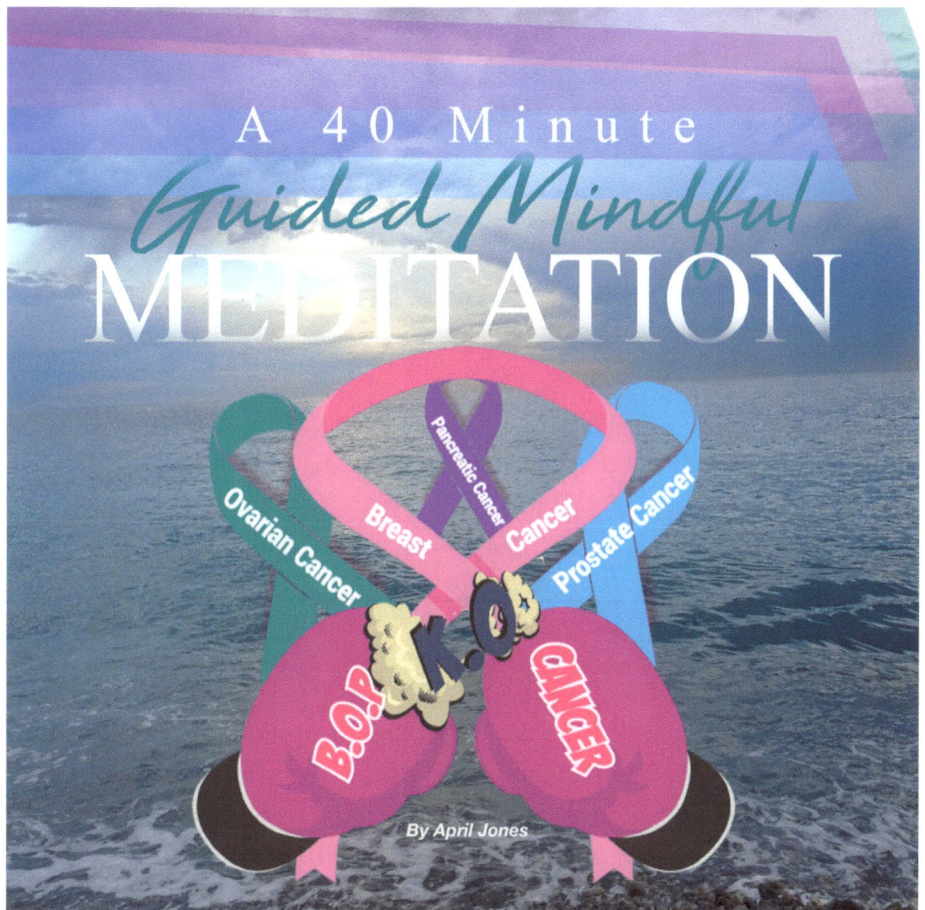

https://store.cdbaby.com/cd/apriljones12

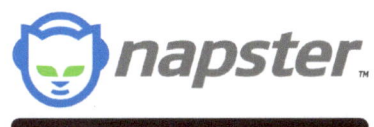
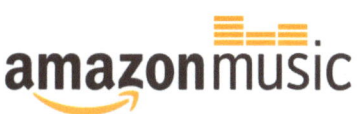

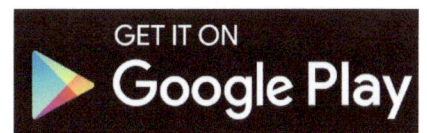

Stronger
IN TIME

You have a fire inside your soul, one that burns brighter as time passes
The clock has finally quit ticking so loud
The once dim flames now ignite with strength and joy for what's to come
Breast cancer was a term used to fight your fire with doubt
Today, the sky shines with possibility and rejoicing hearts
Cancer was what your past used to strengthen your love, your reverence for life
You'll forget the pain, but never the lesson
The fire within your soul burns brighter than ever, and it goes to show
That you've learned to harness the heat, the pressure nonexistent now
You are radiant
Today, you glow with that inner fight and fire
You carry a beautiful, bright hope within your chest
Breast cancer is the ashes that sweep away with your future's promising wind
Your heart is a serene landscape, and the sky is painted with ribbons of pink
Time has passed, and the sky can serve to be a sign of hope for the future
Breathe lighter and exhale the fire
Your encircled love ones warm with the burning embers
They know that you are a beacon of hope, and they too, emit a similar glow
To have fought so hard and come so far, you have a great power
Let the love you cherish envelop you and flower
Cancer could never destroy this newfound serenity, this is certain
Your fire is now closing the curtain
On cancer and its ugly aspects of pain and wounds
You tie a pink ribbon around your arm, you wear it all around
To symbolize this inner fire, to sybolize your mission
To somewhere much more hope-bound

Reflection on my Journey

Reflection on my Journey

www.ingramcontent.com/pod-product-compliance
Lightning Source LLC
Chambersburg PA
CBHW051151220526
45473CB00003B/733